Hope and Help
for the Cancer Patient
A Christian Perspective

By

Dr. Mel Brown

Dedication and Special Thanks

To the Great Physician, the Lord Jesus Christ

To all of the doctors who have taken part in my treatments for cancer, especially Dr. Stewart Garneau, my oncologist, and his staff who provided the finest tender loving care I could have possibly received

To the thousands of people who prayed for my recovery

With great appreciation to these, I dedicate this book.

Mel Brown

Acknowledgments

My wife Barbara who provided encouragement and served as my sounding board and editor

My family members who have supported me in my every endeavor

My church members and friends who have faithfully prayed for me in sickness and health

I couldn't have done it without you!

Hope and Help for the Cancer Patient

A Christian Perspective

Guidance House Publishing

3109 29th Street

Moline, IL 61265

First Edition, 2014

Table of Contents

What Cancer Cannot Do

Cancer is so limited...

It cannot cripple love.

It cannot shatter hope.

It cannot corrode faith.

It cannot eat away peace.

It cannot destroy confidence.

It cannot kill friendship.

It cannot shut out memories.

It cannot silence courage.

It cannot reduce eternal life.

It cannot quench the Spirit.

Author: Unknown

Hope and Help for the Cancer Patient

A Christian Perspective

The Journey Begins

One out of three women and one out of two men will hear their doctor say, "You have cancer." I have heard those words twice in my life, the first time in 1999 with thyroid cancer and the second in 2006 with lymphoma. Realizing that you have cancer is never easy. For most it brings shock, fear and anxiety under the best circumstances. As you listen to the details of the diagnosis and corresponding prognosis, it seems that you have entered a surreal world that is divorced from reality. It is as if the mind is saying, "This can't be happening to me." Nearly every person with whom I've had contact said that upon receiving the news, they thought, "Why me?" This is a perfectly normal response. But in my case, "Why not me?" were the words which immediately flashed through my mind. As a minister and having been at the hospital with many of my members when they first received the diagnosis, I was well aware of how many people get cancer in their lifetime. Although I had provided hope and comfort to a host of people, now I was the one in need of consolation and comfort. Thank God I got it in abundance from both my family and my church members. Having a strong support system will prove to be an immeasurable benefit to any person with cancer.

My first personal experience with cancer was life changing. As I was undergoing a biopsy on my thyroid gland

(A CT scan following an auto accident had revealed the growth.), the doctor mentioned that is was highly unlikely that it was malignant. He added that he did many such biopsies and seldom were they positive for cancer. Imagine my surprise when the doctor called and told me that my biopsy showed that I did have cancer. After undergoing a thyroidectomy, I waited several weeks to receive the radiation treatment which would ablate any remaining cancer. Those weeks of waiting were difficult as the lack of thyroxine made me extremely weak. I was much like a car having no gasoline to power it. When I went into the hospital for the radiation treatment, the room had a stark appearance. There were minimal furnishings in the room. Protective coverings were on everything. There was a paper-covered runway between the bed and the bathroom. I was told that anything I brought into the treatment room would have to be left behind including books, magazines or personal items. They administered a huge radiation capsule which when swallowed felt like a horse pill going down. I had to drink water non-stop and suck on lemon drops constantly to flush the radiation from my salivary glands. The staff came in about every hour to check me with a kind of Geiger counter to see how the radiation was being distributed in my body. I wryly asked the doctor if I would glow in the dark! After 24 hours, I was allowed to go home with the instruction to triple flush the toilet and stay away from my grandchildren. The radiation stayed in my system for several weeks albeit constantly diminishing. That was nearly 15 years ago and my thyroid cancer has not returned. The experience not only drew me much closer to the Lord, it created empathy in my heart for those who suffer, an empathy I hope to exercise the rest of my life.

One's attitude is of primary importance during treatment. Anything that will help you keep a positive attitude will prove to be an invaluable resource. I recommend keeping an *optimal* attitude. This is an attitude which involves avoiding either extreme of the negative or the positive. A Pollyanna attitude refuses to consider the reality of the situation insisting that everything is rosy even when clearly it is not. It is optimistic to the point of foolishness. On the other hand is the negative attitude which is so dark it sees only bad with no hope at all. An optimal attitude grasps the reality and negatives of the situation but also considers the positives and possibilities. It adds the important ingredient of hope. Maintaining an optimal attitude infused with hope will require constant effort during the ups and downs of your treatment. Keep company with people who will lift you up and avoid those naysayers who will drag you down. When you are suffering, well-meaning people can dampen your spirit and damage your attitude with their cancer horror stories and tales of treatment woes. Don't listen to someone going on about how much Uncle Fred suffered or how terrible Aunt Minnie did with her treatment. It will poison your soul. Talk to those who are mental upper-takers not mental undertakers. You want people around you that will make you feel glad they came, not those that will make you feel glad when they go.

It helps to take one day at a time during your treatment. Focus on the day at hand and make the most of it. Some days it will be a full-time task just to get through as unscathed as possible. The Kung Fu Panda got it right when he said, "Yesterday is history, tomorrow is mystery, but today is a gift, that's why they call it the present." Some of your days will be better and some will be worse, but every day will bring you closer to the completion of your treatment.

It helps to maintain a sense of humor whatever the circumstance. The Bible reminds us that a merry heart is like a medicine. If you look for the rose among the thorns instead of the thorn among the roses, it will be medicinal for your spirit. Norman Cousins, who taught for U.C.L.A. School of Medicine and studied the biochemistry of human emotions, suffered from a serious illness which often tended to overwhelm him. When told that he had little chance of surviving, he utilized humor to lift his spirit and improve his symptoms. He watched videos and programs which made him laugh. He soon discovered that his attitude and pain response improved as a result. Ten minutes of genuine belly laughter had an anesthetic effect and afforded him at least two hours of pain-free rest. His story was detailed in the book <u>Anatomy of an Illness</u>, which was also made into a movie.

There are people who become concerned with treatment statistics to the point of obsession and allow a darkened attitude to develop. If the success rate for a particular cancer using a specific treatment is 33%, focus on the fact that one of three will get well and believe that you will be one of them. You can choose to focus on the opposite to your detriment. My father was a heavy smoker for 60 years. Shortly after retirement, he was diagnosed with cancer of the lung. He faced having one lung completely removed followed by months of daily radiation treatments. I recall when he asked his doctor what his chances were, the doctor replied, "Mr. Brown, we don't treat statistics here, we treat patients and we are going to do everything we can to get you well." I knew what the statistics were because

I had looked them up shortly after his diagnosis. He had a 33% chance of living 3 years and an 11% chance for 5 years. Furthermore, after his surgery his doctor told me the cancer had spread to the mediastinum between the lungs and had wrapped around his heart greatly diminishing his chance of successful treatment. He faithfully continued his treatments and focused on the positive that he had the chance and hope of getting well. Our family kept encouraging him with positives and heartening words instead of focusing on the negatives (of which there were many). In spite of the odds, no presence of any cancer was detected through many years of monitoring. He lived more than eight years after his treatment with a good quality of life and died at age 75 from other causes and was still cancer free. Don't allow negative statistics to control your attitude. The Bible says, *As a man thinks in his heart, so he is.*

Treatment of cancer usually involves one of three therapies, surgically removing the malignancy, radiation to burn it out or chemotherapy to poison it. Treatment many involve a combination of these approaches. I experienced treatment with all three methods for my cancers. Cancer treatments currently are producing a 50% cure rate providing a longer and greater quality of life.

One's spiritual life is paramount in importance for overall wellbeing. Prayer and Scripture reading are potent balms for your soul. I continually kept uplifting Scripture verses before me. Jeremiah 29:11 was my promise verse, *I know the plans I have for you says the Lord; plans for good and not evil, to give you a hope and a future*. I placed that Scripture on my desk, bathroom mirror, refrigerator, car and everywhere else I could as a constant reminder. I requested my name be put on as many prayer lists as I could and listened to uplifting sermons and devotions. All proved invaluable during my illness. Spending time in the Psalms and the book of Philippians provided wonderful comfort, faith and hope.

Occasionally, I had to look in the mirror and give myself a good talking to. Those rare confrontations were important attitude adjusters. I lectured myself like a Dutch uncle and never walked away the same after the experience. I also called people on the phone when I knew they would lift me up and provide encouragement. Even a short positive conversation made a big difference to me.

We are fortunate to be living in the age where newer and better medicines are not only being used to kill the cancer cells but alleviate the side effects as well. I recall meeting a fellow patient undergoing chemotherapy as I was starting my treatments. She had been successfully treated for a different kind of cancer with chemotherapy 20 years before and mentioned that they didn't have the wonderful drugs back then to control nausea. She assured me that I should be grateful for the progress and keep that in mind as I dealt with side effects. I did, and it helped me to consider how much worse it would have been without the resources now available to me.

It is helpful to remember these advantages we now have as cancer patients: improved knowledge of the many forms of cancer, better medical facilities for treatment, better tools for diagnosis and treatment, competent specialists treating all forms of cancer and effective medicines for treatment of the disease and control of side effects.

During my 50 years of ministry, I have encountered hundreds of cancer sufferers and have seen remarkable progress made in some of their treatments. During the last several years, I have watched many women go through treatment for breast cancer, and I can't think of a single one who has not done well. That is a great catalyst for hope.

Here are additional suggestions to consider as you fight your battle against cancer.

1. Ask others for whatever assistance you may need. Enlist the help of close friends and relatives to drive you to appointments, help with chores, babysit your children, listen to your concerns, assist you with meals, run interference with financial matters or insurance issues, accompany you to church and provide personal support. Remember people are not mind readers and will not automatically know your needs. We are exhorted in Galatians 6:2 to bear one another's burdens. This necessitates allowing others to be our burden bearers.

2. If you are going through chemotherapy, it is wise to have another person with you when you see the doctor. However good your memory may have been before chemotherapy, you may develop "chemo brain" and your memory becomes impaired. I always took my wife to my appointments and later when we were discussing what the doctor had said, I realized I missed much of that conversation. That was especially difficult for me because I had such an excellent memory before I began therapy.

3. Build into your life as many uplifting things as you reasonably can each day. These may include telephone calls to friends, a little handcraft, brows-

ing through old photos, a drive in the car, etc. These things will help to counteract your tendency toward depression. If you find yourself getting seriously depressed, inform your doctor so s/he can properly administer treatment or get you the help you require.

4. Talk out your fears and worries with an empathetic listener with whom you are comfortable, and don't bottle up your concerns and feelings.

5. Diet and nutrition are important elements in the treatment of any illness, but often during cancer treatment, eating a healthy diet is difficult due to irritation of the digestive system. My doctor's treatment room was stocked with Ensure which provides essential nutrients needed when regular food is impossible to tolerate. Try ice-cold or frozen Ensure supplements or milk shakes. Note that during chemo, many become lactose intolerant and cannot drink milk products, but shakes from McDonalds do not contain lactose. It always pays to follow a healthy diet but especially when fighting a serious illness. Find the foods which you can tolerate best (or tolerate at all) and build your diet around them. In times when I was the sickest, I could only eat noodles or scrambled eggs. Fortunately, I was able to tolerate those foods when I couldn't eat anything else. A competent nutritionist can offer helpful advice.

6. Plan how you will spend the treatment sessions. Consider enjoyable diversional activities

such as doing crafts, puzzles, reading, journaling, watching TV or videos, using electronic devices, visiting or resting. When the mind is pleasurably occupied, mood is elevated and pain and discomfort are decreased. I found I could handle the chemotherapy sessions best when my daughter and four-year-old granddaughter accompanied me. We talked, munched, played simple games, watched programs and read together during my sessions. Being so occupied, it made time pass faster, gave me an emotional boost and made the sessions more bearable, especially the long ones.

7. Television can provide many kinds of entertainment and diversion. My children bought me a television for my bedroom, but I soon learned that some programs tended to pull me down and others lifted me up. During my first round of chemotherapy, I tried to watch a medical program but it was depressing and I had to quickly change the channel to lighter fare. Inspiring and humorous shows worked best for me but only in short doses.

8. Don't allow yourself to get overtired. When you need rest, take it. Your strength will become depleted as therapy progresses and you will need adequate rest to conserve your energy and recharge your battery.

9. Music therapy is used to assist patients with their mental and emotional health with great success. Listening to music usually has a positive effect on your emotions. Try various types of music and see what works for you.

10. Work to keep the stressors in your life at a minimum. Undergoing cancer treatment is stressful enough without allowing problematic things to needlessly add to your stress level. My associates at work ran interference for me and handled things which would have potentially overwhelmed me. My wife and children did the same for me at home. Minimalizing stress and hostility can make a marked difference in your recovery.

11. Don't delay calling your doctor or going to the emergency room if you become very sick. I spiked a high temperature in the middle of the night as I had developed a serious infection and went immediately to the emergency room for treatment. Delay of treatment is unwise since the immune system is already compromised.

12. It may be necessary to restrict visitors while undergoing treatment. I found talking could drain my energy quickly, so I reserved my visiting mainly for family members. When I felt too tired, I simply said I needed to rest and did so. My daughter made sure that I saw my granddaughter nearly every day but never let the visits overtire me.

13. Don't hesitate to ask people to pray for you. My name was put on many prayer lists for which I was thankful. I was uplifted and blessed when people wrote me notes or sent me cards, especially those with personal messages. I read and reread them and appreciated the encouragement and personal concern.

14. Participate in a web site such as caringbridge.org for sharing experiences with others and allowing them to share with you. It can be a wonderful source of communication, encouragement and spiritual connection with others.

15. Search out the stories and testimonies of those who have been overcomers. Their personal stories will inspire and encourage you. Numerous articles and books can be found online and in stores that tell the stories of people just like you who struggled through and overcame their illnesses.

16. Maintain your inner strength through dwelling on the meaningful things and purpose in your life. These are the things we live for, the reasons we have to live and the things that matter most to us, e.g., our family, our faith, our friends, our unfinished plans and dreams. Someone wryly said, "They say we will not leave this earth until our work is done, so I'm going to be around for a long time because I'm so far behind, it will take forever for me to catch up."

17. Try to maintain physical strength with some kind of light exercise. Even walking a few minutes increases circulation and improves all the body functions.

18. Rely on your faith in the Lord and His presence to see you through the tough times. He is our ever present help in time of trouble and promises to never leave us or forsake us. He is always only a prayer away! My family doctor tells his cancer patients to stay in church as it can provide you with faith, hope

and love, all of which are precious commodities during times of distress.

19. You can will yourself to accomplish amazing things through the thinking processes. This is commonly referred to as the mind-body connection. Fill your mind with things that are lovely, pure, true, honest and of good report and meditate on these things (Philippians 4:8). I have seen people intensely focus their mind so that they have been able to paralyze muscles and restrict pain. Biofeedback and hypnosis, even without a trance, can allow the mind to do amazing things for the body.

20. Accept that there will be ups and downs during your cancer journey. Ecclesiastes gives some good advice in dealing with these vacillating times, *In the day of prosperity rejoice and in the day of adversity consider, God has set the one over against the other.* Appreciate and enjoy the better days and remember and anticipate them during the bad ones. Some have found comfort during especially bad times by dwelling on the thought, "This too shall pass."

I recall my first visit with the oncologist as he discussed what I should expect during treatment for my malignancy. He used a vivid word picture which I would cling to throughout the course of my treatment. He said, "Pastor, it as if you are entering a long black tunnel which is filled with large rocks. Some of which are huge boulders. But there is light at the end of the tunnel. My job is to pull you through, get you over the rocks and bring you safely to the other side." Many times when I was stuck on a rock in that dark tunnel, I pictured him pulling me through and kept anticipating getting to the light at the end.

My chemotherapy consisted of infusions with five different drugs, five days in a row, every three weeks. The week of treatments and the following week were the roughest. The third week provided several days of relief and recuperation. I decided to write a weekly blog to share with my friends and fellow church members. I was able to express what I was going through, my thoughts, my feelings and could provide updates on my progress. These blogs have since been read by others who have gone through cancer treatment. Many have shared how much they were helped by reading them as they went through their own dark tunnel. I have included them in this book with the hope that they will uplift and encourage you in your journey through your treatment regimentation. Following the blogs, I have provided a list of helpful suggestions, some important and practical lessons from God's Word about our suffering and the personal stories of cancer survivors which have been an encouragement to me during my two bouts with cancer. I hope they will do the same for you.

The Blogs
(July 1st through May 12th)

July 1st

It is Saturday morning. I have just completed my first week of treatment. On the first day of treatment, I suffered a reaction to the chemo drugs administered. I experienced a rash on my upper body and the doctor immediately addressed the problem. After giving me a drug to counteract the reaction, he slowed the drip of the IV. Although it extended the time of the treatment, I had no further problem. But I remember thinking, "What if I have a more serious reaction or can't tolerate this drug at all?" Since it was my first exposure to chemo, it did not get me off to a very good start and left me concerned about future treatments and how my body would react. It turned out to be a session of nearly eight hours after which I was totally exhausted. It made me very apprehensive about the other four drugs which were yet to be administered during the next several days. Fortunately, as I was exiting the office, I encountered a nurse whom I had counseled years before. She stopped to give me a hug and gave me many encouraging words as to how I had influenced her life and family. It was just what I needed to lift my spirits. Isn't it amazing how God brings what you need into your life just when you need it. From that incident came an appropriate and necessary prayer during the weeks of treatment, "Lord give me what I need, when I need it, Amen."

The nausea is being handled well with meds and I'm dealing trial and error with the fatigue factor. I tend to have more energy early in the morning and try to make the most of it in those earliest hours. I am scheduled for my next week of treatment the week of July 10th. Barb has been my personal nurse and has taken very good care of me. Thank you for your prayers, cards and notes of encouragement - they mean more to me than you will ever know. It is great to be part of such a loving caring church family. On a final note, someone said, "When you start to lose your hair, will you part it on the left or the right?" and I thought, *neither because it will be departed.* Thanks again for your faithful prayers and concern.

July 8th

I will plan on updating this blog every Saturday morning to let you know how things are going. This has been a good week with my strength gradually increasing. If all goes well, I plan to be in church and preach the sermon on "Careful Instead of Care-full Living" tomorrow morning. Thank you for your continuing prayers and demonstrations of concern, I so appreciate each one. I begin my next round of treatment on Monday morning. Lord willing, I'll see you all tomorrow.

July 10th

Unfortunately I underestimated how weak the chemo would leave me. I was sitting in my office on Sunday morning getting ready to preach but feeling weak and tired. When I got up to walk into the sanctuary, I stood, took two steps and barely made it back to the chair. I was woozy and felt utter fatigue. I knew there was no way I would be able to walk to the pulpit much less be able to preach. I told the associate pastor he was on and didn't move from the chair for the next half hour. My wife then drove me home and I spent the rest of the day in bed. The chemo has left my intestinal tract feeling raw and I'm totally zapped of strength. I will not underestimate its effects on my energy level the immediate days after therapy in the future. When my strength is failing, it is a good time to meditate on Isaiah 34:21, *They that wait upon the Lord shall renew their strength, they shall mount up with wings as eagles; they shall run and not be weary; they shall walk and not faint.* This verse refers to the eagle growing weak and having trouble flying because his feathers are failing. But as he patiently waits for moulting to occur wherein his feathers are replaced, he finds new strength and can soar once again. I'm like the eagle and look forward to regaining my strength as the effects of the chemo wear off. I trust the Lord that my strength will return. Also since my hair came out in bunches I feel like I'm without feathers!

July 15ᵗʰ

It is 5:00 a.m. Saturday and I'm in my study at home providing this weekly update. I completed my second round of treatment yesterday which went well. After having gone through the first round, I made some adjustments in diet, medicines and schedule to better tolerate the process and it has been helpful. One change involves avoiding sick people. If we have staff sickness going around the church office, I go in early in the morning when no one is there and leave before everyone else arrives. Other changes include minimizing stress as much as possible and focusing on my goal of getting well. I look at each session of treatment as a round in a fight for which I need to prepare. Then surviving its bruises, I prepare for the next round. I know I have four invaluable resources through this process:

(1) The constant presence of the Great Physician, the Lord Jesus Christ, who promised He will never leave us nor

forsake us and always understands our every feeling and circumstance

(2) The finest of medical care I could ever receive to pull me through this dark tunnel over the boulders and out into the light

(3) The strong encouragement and support from the finest church family I could ever have, all who pray for me, offer comforting support through cards, uplifting notes and verses, and are regularly encouraging me

(4) Incredibly supportive family members who are always there when I need them (Barb, my faithful private duty nurse is always "on call" in the Brown residence; daughter Lori, on summer break from her teaching duties, joins me during my chemo sessions. We enjoy this sweet personal time together. She also sees that I get regular visits with her daughter Kaitlynn who brightens up any day. Daughter Cheryl comes with her family periodically on weekends from Chicago and calls regularly to see if I need anything. Those visits with her three children, Maelynn, Ryan and Brendan, give me great joy and something to look forward to. Son Tim comes from Morrison a couple times a week to help with some of my chores. During his visits, we enjoy wonderful times of sharing and fellowship).

Well, I now have no hair, I'm as bald as a cue ball. If I walked around with a lollipop in my mouth, I could pass for Kojak or if I put a ring in my ear, I could pass for Mr. Clean. Wait till you see me in my new hat! Meantime, I'm trying to decide between the Elvis wig and the Ted Koppel look for my new hairpiece - relax, I'm just kidding.

I'll miss tomorrow's services but, Lord willing, I'll speak

the next Sunday.

With much love and appreciation

July 22nd

Good Morning

This is the end of the second week following my second round of therapy. It has been a precarious week characterized by low white blood cell counts, tiredness and occasionally a little wooziness (now there's a technical medical term for you). The meds are controlling nausea fairly well. But one night I awakened with severe nausea and immediately put an anti-nausea medicine under my tongue to prevent severe vomiting. I'm glad that the various antiemetic drugs are available to control the nausea. My doctor has given me three kinds of anti-nausea drugs, each more powerful than the other. If one doesn't control it, I can try another to get the job done.

I'm also learning to adjust to the other complications. I'm pacing myself, not overtaxing my energy levels to cope with the tiredness. I'm trying to avoid pathogens (germs) whenever possible (You should see me run when someone sneezes or coughs.) and standing and moving slowly to handle the orthostatic hypotension (wooziness). All things considered, it has not been too bad a week and I have much for which to be thankful.

My daughters and their families have been on vacation together in Florida for the last week or so. I've missed them so much, but I've appreciated the many e-mails, pictures and phone calls while they have been gone. I eagerly anticipate their return on Monday. Tim came last night to finish a couple of chores for me. We talked and watched a movie (comedy) together which is always enjoyable. Barb faithfully fulfills her role as my private-duty nurse, but her overtime pay is killing me. (How much bowing and scraping can one stand?) I appreciate how many of you at Edgewood have been faithful in your prayers for me. I've learned that you have added me to numerous prayer lists be they friends, churches, or other groups. Again the cards, notes and words of encouragement have been so important.

I have chosen the book of Philippians as my focus during this ordeal. I read it over and over, claim its many promises, attempt to follow its many principles and turn its words of wisdom into prayers and personal petitions. Its valuable themes are how to have joy in spite of difficult circumstances, God working in spite of and through our circumstances, the example of Christ through His suffering, the constant need for attitude adjustment to see things from God's perspective instead of our own narrow focus, the importance of turning our worries into expressions of concern and prayer requests to God and the all-important principle of always practicing positive Christ-like thinking. These have been powerful daily helps for me. I remember that WITH MAN ALONE, many things are *impossible*, but WITH GOD, all things are *possible* (Matthew 19:26). Lord willing, I will speak a week from Sunday on Philippians chapter four, part two of the message, "Careful Instead of Care-full Living."
Please continue to pray for my healing, strength and complication-free recovery.

July 29th

I've had a good week in spite of fighting a cold and cough. I'm gradually adjusting to seeing myself with no hair. Out of habit when I get out of the shower every morning, I still find myself reaching for the hair brush. Then I look in the mirror and think, "You won't be needing that." Now all this has led to another potential problem - the bugs think my head is their personal landing strip. Maybe I'll have to "grease the skids" so they will slide right on off! I mention it so when you see me tomorrow, you won't be shocked by my changed appearance. I've had a good energy level this week and have succeeded in getting a lot done.

I thought you would appreciate reading these recent comments from Rick Warren, author of The *Purpose Driven Life* whose wife recently went through her second bout with cancer and became acutely ill during the treatment. This article has been a source of blessing to me and I hope will be to you also.

People ask me, what is the purpose of life? And I respond: In a nutshell, life is preparation for eternity. We were made to last forever and God wants us to be with Him in Heaven. One day my heart is going to stop, and that will be the end of my body - but not the end of me. I may live 60 to 100 years on earth, but I am going to spend trillions of years in eternity. This is the warm-up act - the dress rehearsal. God wants us to practice on earth what we will do forever in eternity. We were made by God and for God, and until you figure that out, life isn't going to make sense. Life is a series of problems: Either you are in one now, you're just coming out of one or you're getting ready to go into another one. The reason for this is that God is more interested in your character than your comfort. God is more interested in making your life holy than He is in making your life happy. We can be reasonably happy here on earth, but that's not the goal of life. The goal is to grow in character, in Christ likeness. This past year has been the greatest year of my life but also the toughest, with my wife, Kay, getting cancer. I used to think that life was hills and valleys - you go through a dark time, then you go to the mountaintop, back and forth. I don't believe that anymore. Rather than life being hills and valleys, I believe that it's kind of like two rails on a railroad track, and at all times you have something good and something bad in your life. No matter how good things are in your life, there is always something bad that needs to be worked on. And no matter how bad things are in your life, there is always something good you can thank God for. You can focus on your purposes, or you can focus on your problems. If you focus on your problems, you're going into self-centeredness, "which is my problem, my issues, my pain." But one of the easiest ways to get rid of pain is to get your focus off yourself and onto God and others. We discovered quickly that in spite of the prayers of hundreds of thousands of people, God was not going to heal Kay or make it easy for her. It has been very difficult for her, and yet God has strengthened her character, given her a ministry of helping other people, given her a testimony, drawn her closer to Him and to people. You have to learn to deal with both the good and the bad of life. Actually, sometimes learning to deal with the good is harder. For instance, this past year, all of a sudden, when the book sold 15 million copies, it made me instantly very wealthy. It also brought a lot of notoriety that I had never had to deal with before. I don't think God gives you money or notoriety for your own ego or for you to live a life of ease. So I began to ask God what He wanted me to do with this money, notoriety and influence. He gave me two different passages that helped me decide what to do, II Corinthians 9 and Psalm 72. First, in spite of all the money coming in, we would not change our lifestyle one bit. We made no major purchases. Second, about midway through last year, I stopped taking a salary from the church. Third, we set up foundations to fund an initiative we call 'The Peace Plan' to plant churches, equip leaders, assist the poor, care for the sick, and educate the next generation. Fourth, I added up all that the church had paid me in the 24 years since I started the church, and I gave it all back. It was liberating to be able to serve God for free. We need to ask ourselves: Am I going to live for possessions? Popularity? Am I going to be driven by pressures? Guilt? Bitterness? Materialism? Or am I going to be driven by God's purposes (for my life)? When I get up in the morning, I sit on the side of my bed and say, God, if I don't get anything else done today, I want to know You more and love You better. God didn't put me on earth just to fulfill a to-do list. He's more interested in what I am than what I do. That's why we're called human beings, not human doings. Happy moments, PRAISE GOD. Difficult moments, SEEK GOD. Quiet moments, WORSHIP GOD. Painful moments, TRUST GOD. Every moment, THANK GOD.

Lord willing, I plan to preach "Careful Instead of Carefull Living" Part 2 tomorrow morning. I will begin my third week of treatment on Monday. Thank you so much for your love, prayers, concern, cards and notes. I am very appreciative of each one. Lord willing, I'll see you tomorrow.

August 5th

This week I completed my third series of treatments which went very well. Additionally, I received a very encouraging report from my latest PET scan which showed that the treatment is working well to kill the cancer. Now we have

28

to finish the job! As my doctor says, "Our goal isn't to get you to 3rd base but to hit a home run." Later this month, I am going to the University of Nebraska Medical Center for a consultation with a leading lymphoma expert. He will review all of my records and recommend any other measures that may be taken for maximum benefit. Although my treatment is going well, it will be good to ensure that we are leaving no stone unturned in facilitating my recovery. It was good to be in the pulpit last Sunday and finish the two-part message on "Careful Instead of Care-full Living." There has been an overwhelming response from so many about the benefit of those messages. Clearly, lots of us struggle with stress in our lives. Thank God we are "in Christ" and have "Christ in us" providing strength and help. Besides His presence we have His written word to give us guidance for life's struggles and problems. We ran out of the handouts at the information desk in the foyer although we printed a large supply. We have restocked the supply and should have plenty of the several handouts for "Six Practices of Successful Families," and the two latest handouts on, "Careful Instead of Care-full Living."

A touch of humor here – hope this is never true of me! A country church held a potluck supper on opening night of a revival series. The guest speaker was invited to lead the food line, but he declined saying, "I can't eat a big meal before I preach. It detracts from my ability to deliver a good sermon." Two hours later, several women were cleaning up the church kitchen, when one declared, "I believe that preacher might as well have eaten his fill at suppertime."

I have so enjoyed your cards and notes. They have touched and blessed me so much. Your faithfulness in praying for me has been a great contribution toward recovering my health and strength. Finally, I leave you with one of my favorite Scriptures and a couple of additional thoughts.

For I know the plans I have for you says the Lord. They are plans for good and not for evil, to give you a hope and a future (Jeremiah 29:11).

Food for thought:
"An impossibility is something no one can do until someone does it." "A hospital is a place to wind up people who are run down." "Opportunity is something that knocks but doesn't turn the door handle." And a little humorous one: "An optimist is a mail carrier who enjoys the view when treed by a dog." **Remember, "God is the God of the impossible."**
Thank you for caring. Lord willing, I'll be preaching on August 20th and 27th.

August 12th

This week concludes the 2nd of my three-week treatment cycle. This is the week of special vulnerability to fatigue, weakness and infection. It has been a reasonably good week and I am looking forward to next week when there is usually marked improvement, strengthening and sense of wellbeing. By the grace of God, I work on avoiding thinking about the "what ifs" during this process. 2 Timothy 1:7 says, *For God has not given us a spirit of fear, but of power and of love and of a sound mind.* As I am fond of saying, fear stands for **F**anaticized **E**xperiences **A**ppearing **R**eal or in other words, the imagined "what ifs" that intrude on our minds. No wonder God so often counsels to *fear not* in His Word. In 2 Timothy, He gives the antidote to fear. It is the spirit (attitude) of power, love and a sound mind. All three

of these qualities are given to us by the Holy Spirit of God (Gal. 5:22, 23, 1 John 4:18, 1 Cor. 2:4). The sound mind means self-control, discipline, restoring to one's senses. It is one thing to have genuine fear and to work through it or act in spite of it, but it is an entirely different matter to have fear conjured up by an overactive imagination filled with "what ifs". The Spirit of God provides the source of both reality checks and attitude adjustments toward strength, love and restoring us to our senses - that is a sound mind. A good example of that process is the testimony of Kay Warren, Rick Warren's wife, whom I mentioned in a recent blog. Through her experience she sought God's answer to the question not so much as to "why me" but "why now"? Her suffering opened her eyes to other's suffering and became a purpose-driven experience for her and produced a profound change in her life. You can see God's work in her life through the process. Here are some brief excerpts from her testimony. (*LAKE FOREST, Calif. BP)*
Kay Warren has an impressive ministry resume. She's the wife of Rick Warren, perhaps America's best-known pastor. She's a Bible teacher and the president of Acts of Mercy, a foundation she and Rick established to help vulnerable people and needy communities. But she admits there are some things about God she just doesn't understand. Suffering tops that list. God opened Kay's heart to suffering in March 2002. She was at home, reading through a news-magazine, when she saw an article with photographs of Africans suffering with AIDS - images so horrifying she had to cover her eyes. One line of text said, "12 million children orphaned in Africa due to AIDS." "That was a shocking statistic to me. I couldn't believe there were 12 million orphans anywhere due to anything," Kay says. The number –12 million – continued to haunt her. She told God,

"Well, even if it's true, there's nothing I can do about it. I'm a white, suburban, soccer-mom type person. This has nothing to do with me." When the thought of so much suffering was still with her a month later, she realized she had come to a crossroads. NO LONGER A NUMBER" I made a conscious decision to open my heart to the pain," she says. "When I did, God broke my heart. He shattered it in a million pieces, and I cried for days." I knew I couldn't stand before God when He called me home and look Him in the face and tell Him, 'Yes, I knew about the suffering of millions of people, but I did nothing about it,'" she says. Kay began sharing her heart with Rick, who encouraged her but insisted God was speaking to her - not to him or to their congregation at Saddleback Church. Kay began reading about AIDS/HIV and talking with experts. She was deeply moved by the testimony of Bruce Wilkinson, author of "The Prayer of Jabez," and his wife, Darlene Marie, who moved to South Africa to serve the poor. But it was a trip to Malawi that transformed her heart. At one house, she met a 15-year-old boy who was raising his 11-year-old brother and 3-year-old sister. Their parents had died from AIDS. Kay's voice breaks as she recalls holding the little girl outside the hut: "She has no daddy to stand proudly when she marries, no mama to answer her cries in the middle of the night when she's had a bad dream, no mom to tell her how to be a woman." On that trip, 12 million ceased to be a number. It turned into faces and names." That's the only way we'll ever be moved to do anything about the pandemic - when we move it beyond statistics and it becomes personal," Kay says. "Each of those I was holding and weeping for, God is weeping for." A VISION DISRUPTED Rick came along on Kay's second trip to Africa. Up to that point, he was thinking more about the Great Commission

in Matthew 28:19-20 - building his church and strengthening pastors around the world - than helping the poor and needy by fulfilling the Great Commandment of Matthew 22:37-40. During Rick's first five hours on African soil, though, God captured his heart for the world's suffering and began showing him what to do about it. On that trip, the P.E.A.C.E. Plan - attacking the world's giants of spiritual darkness, lack of servant leaders, poverty, disease, and ignorance - was born. They began working to put the P.E.A.C.E. Plan into motion - and then Kay was diagnosed with breast cancer. "Breast cancer seemed at the time like the biggest interruption," Kay says. And though she never asked, "Why me?" she did ask, "Why now?" When she became very sick during chemotherapy, Rick also had to pull back from ministry, and the P.E.A.C.E. Plan practically halted for several months. They both asked, "What is this about, God?" What it was about was increasing her empathy for people who suffer. Her hair was just growing back after chemotherapy in July 2004 when she traveled to Thailand for an international AIDS conference. She visited a widow who had AIDS and listened as she talked about how sick her medicine made her. When Kay told her about the medicine that made her hair fall out, each woman found a friend who understood her suffering. Witnessing - and experiencing - suffering have made God both more intimate to her and more mysterious, she says. She understands more about Him - and less. "I don't get this world system," she says. "I don't get the suffering." In Rwanda, she saw churches that had been used as slaughterhouses and skulls stacked on top of each other with evidence of machete wounds. In Cambodia, she heard of people killing each other in horrible ways. Around the world she's seen countless orphans. "When you see suffering, it takes your heart and wrenches it," she said. "It has made me long for [Jesus'] appearing. It has made me long for suffering to come to an end." What she does understand more than ever is how, as a Christian, she takes God's presence with her wherever she goes. CHRIST'S HANDS "When I go into a place - whether it's a hospital or mud hut or Mother Teresa's home for the dying - I take His presence and I offer it," she says. "I'm His reflection ... His messenger ... His hands. That's very intimate." Kay is convinced that the church is the answer to the world's global giants, like AIDS. "The evangelical church has been asleep at the wheel," she says. "We have been absent from our post in caring for people and their needs for a very long time now. But I see repentance happening. I see people waking up with the same shock that I did and wanting to respond. That fills me with hope." Kay knows the world won't be perfect until Jesus returns. "But we can push back the darkness," she says. "We can bring His presence and His light. We can be His hands that relieve the suffering, that comfort the dying, that care for the sick. God is mobilizing His people to touch broken and hurting people with His love," she says.

Clearly through the dark days of her second bout with cancer, God provided an amazing light of revelation for her. As recorded in the Gospels, Jesus spent 55% of His time ministering to the sick. His example speaks for itself. We can make a difference in people's lives, one life at a time - Jesus did!

I'm doing very well by the grace of God and I'm so grateful to Him and for all of you. Your prayers and support have sustained me again and again (Phil. 1:3-8).
Like Kay Warren I don't ask "why me" but know that He

knows the "why" because there is a time to every purpose under heaven (Ecclesiastes 3:1).

Lord willing, I will preach the last two Sundays of August. On a lighter note, I'm not only getting used to seeing myself bald but actually kind of liking it - a sure sign that I have either come to my senses or ...

August 19th

This is the third week of my treatment cycle and normally I would be getting ready for my next round of chemo, but because I am going to Nebraska for a consultation the end of this month, I have a brief respite from my treatment cycle. For that reason, I should be able to be in the pulpit both tomorrow and next Sunday barring any unforeseen complications. I eagerly anticipate and enjoy each opportunity to preach. This fall we will begin a new round of 20-20 groups studying *The Normal Christian Life* (studies in Romans), *Sit, Walk, Stand* (studies in Ephesians) and *Be Joyful* (studies in Philippians). These studies are so vital to the understanding and appreciation of victorious Christian living, I am encouraging every one of our people to participate in these studies. Details will be announced for the various groups starting in early September.

Watchman Nee, whose prolific ministry led to the writing of the *Normal Christian Life*, was responsible for starting more than 200 churches. He spent the final 20 years of his life imprisoned by the communists because of his faith and his refusal to stop preaching the uncompromised message of Jesus Christ. He certainly experienced persecution, hardship and enormous pressures in his life, yet he remained steadfast in his faith and walk. He wrote these inspiring words of encouragement and insight for us. *God ... made us to sit with Him in heavenly places, in Christ Je-*

sus (Eph. 2:6). What does it really mean to sit down? When we walk or stand we bear on our legs all the weight of our own body, whereas when we sit down our entire weight rests upon the chair or bench upon which we sit. We grow weary when we walk or stand, but we feel rested when we sit down for a while. In walking or standing we expend a great deal of energy, but when we are seated we relax at once because the strain no longer falls upon our muscles and sinews but upon something outside of ourselves. So too in spiritual things, to sit down is simply to rest our whole weight - our load, ourselves, our future, everything - upon the Lord. We let Him bear the responsibility and cease to carry it ourselves.

What a perfect commentary on the verse, *Casting all your care upon Him, for He cares for you* (1 Peter 5:7). Note that we are to cast *ALL* of our care upon Him because He cares for us. For most of us, this is easier said than done, especially on a continuing basis. Nee goes on with his exposition and uses this illustration. *The temptation to try is ingrained in human nature. Let me tell you something I have seen in my own country at the salt pits. In China some coolies can carry a load of salt weighing 120 kilos; others as much as 250 kilos. Now along comes a man who can only carry 120 kilos and here is a load of 250 kilos. He knows perfectly well it is far too heavy for him, but although he cannot possibly carry it, he still tries. As a youngster I used to amuse myself watching ten or twenty of these fellows come along and try, though every one of them knew he could not possibly manage it. In the end he must give up and make way for the one who could. How often is it only at the point of utter despair with ourselves that we remember the Lord and relinquish to Him the task He is so ready and able to perform! The sooner we do so the better, for while we monopolize it we leave little room for the Spirit's mighty working.* This example also illustrates the application of the verse, *Apart from me you can do nothing* (John 15:5).

Ultimately, the secret of burden bearing is transferring the burden to the Lord in much the same way we would transfer a heavy bag to be carried by a baggage handler at an airport and then watch as he carries it away. The transfer can only be accomplished if we yield the heavy bag to him and his control. What cares and burdens are you carrying instead of giving them over to the Lord Jesus to carry for you? I'll see you from the pulpit tomorrow, Lord willing, when I preach the sermon entitled, "Seek to Be Meek Instead of Weak." As ever, I am so appreciative of your thoughts, prayers and expressions of love and concern.

August 26th

I have enjoyed a very good week with a reprieve from chemo so I can travel to Nebraska next week without being sick. I'll resume my chemo after I return from Omaha. With the many notes and cards I have recently received, you have included Scripture quotations which have been a special blessing to you or which you thought would have a special application for me. I have enjoyed and appreciated every one of them. One of our ladies who recently went through a serious illness took the time to share the verses that kept her spirit up throughout her ordeal. I have used numerous Scriptures in the same way and have also used the many you have quoted to me in recent weeks. Here are a few of those treasured verses:

Be merciful to me, O God, be merciful to me! For my soul trusts in You; And in the shadow of Your wings I will make my refuge, Until these calamities have passed by. I will cry out to God Most High, To God who performs all things for me (Psalm 57:1-2).

I have set the LORD always before me; Because He is at my right hand I shall not be moved. Therefore my heart is glad, and my glory rejoices; My flesh also will rest in hope (Psalm 16:8-9). *Then shall your light break forth as the morning, and thine health shall spring forth speedily: and your righteousness shall go before you; the glory of the LORD shall be your rear guard* (Isaiah 58:8).

For I, the LORD your God, will hold your right hand, Saying to you, Fear not I will help you (Isaiah 41:13).

Now to Him who is able to do exceedingly abundantly above all that we ask or think, according to the power that works in us (Ephesians 3:20).

Blessed is he who considers the poor; The LORD will deliver him in time of trouble (Psalm 41:1).

God is our refuge and strength, A very present help in trouble (Psalm 46:1).

The eyes of the LORD are on the righteous, And His ears are open to their cry. The righteous cry out, and the LORD hears, And delivers them out of all their troubles (Psalm 34:15, 17).

But those who wait on the LORD shall renew their strength; they shall mount up with wings like eagles, they shall run and not be weary, they shall walk and not faint (Isaiah 40:31).

That I may know Him and the power of His resurrection and the fellowship of His sufferings, being made conformable unto His death (Philippians 3:10).

Most of us would like to have the power of His resurrection in our lives, but we want to avoid the second part of the verse, the fellowship of His sufferings; yet they are clearly linked together. The power of His resurrection and fellowship of His sufferings are part of being made conformable unto His death, which is dying to self that there may be more of Christ and his power operating and flowing in and through us. Ultimately, it is about having less of self and more of Christ possessing and influencing every area of our lives. Also, going through hardships truly creates understanding and empathy toward others who are going through similar hardships in their lives; hence the saying about Jesus that He is a high priest who can be touched with the feelings of our infirmities (Hebrews 4:15).

Lord willing, I will be preaching tomorrow morning on the subject, "What It Means to Be Blessed. " I can hardly wait to preach that message and see you all then.

September 2nd

Good Morning on this beautiful Saturday. I arrived home from Omaha, Nebraska about 8:00 p.m. yesterday evening after being evaluated at the University of Nebraska Medical Center last Thursday. When I was there, the doctor told me he had some things he wanted to say to me before we discussed the details of my medical condition. He began by saying, "You have cancer and I know you've experienced some changes because of it. Life is more precious to you because you are more aware of its potential brevity. Things you took for granted now mean more to you because you realize how quickly and easily you could lose them. Your priorities have been reordered with things which seemed so important before now being far less important and things which before were more trivial are now far more important. Things you previously took for granted, you now savor, isn't that true?" When I responded that all he said was true, he added, "When you get well, never lose the lessons your bout with cancer have taught you, and you will be richer for it always." I will remember that sage advice. The school of cancer can teach us many wise lessons about life and living as well as what is really important.

Overall the trip went very well. After reviewing my biopsy slides, CT and PET scans and other pertinent reports, he examined me and evaluated my condition and treatment progress. His conclusion was that my treatment is proceeding well and the prognosis is very positive with a high probability of complete remission. In a nutshell, my treatment is on target and we should stay the course. He answered my questions and discussed further treatment and monitoring after chemo is completed. It was an excellent session. I handled the trip as well as I could have expected and was accompanied by Barbara, my daughter Lori and granddaughter Kaitlynn which made the trip much more enjoyable than it might have been. I thank the Lord for my progress as I have reached the half-way point in my chemotherapy and request that you continue to faithfully pray for me that God will restore me to health and strength and that future treatments will go well. I cannot thank you enough nor express all of my appreciation for your love, care, concern and especially your many prayers on my behalf. I resume my chemotherapy next week for my fourth session of treatment.

It is early on Saturday morning and the early-hour writing is the result of my sleeplessness. This week marked the completion of my fourth chemotherapy treatment cycle. The treatment regimentation which I completed yesterday went well although I began with a sinus infection which was treated early in the week and is improving. I am grateful for the progress and relief. I continue to feel the unflagging support and benefit of your faithful prayers on my behalf. This together with the fruit of the Spirit, i.e., love, joy, peace, long-suffering, gentleness, goodness, meekness, self-control and faith, made available through being "in Christ" and having "Christ in me," are a great source of encouragement to me. It is not my peace I need, but Christ's peace flowing in and through me. Did you notice the extent of Christ's peace when He was alive on earth? He slept through a powerful storm while on a small boat. On the night before going to Calvary, when betrayed, arrested, deserted, denied, falsely accused and abused, He displayed an amazing inward peace. He referred to this peace as *my peace* and said, *my peace I give unto you.* Since Christ is in us, that same peace He had is readily available to us at all times. In our lives we may experience many troubles, but His peace is always available to us if we will only depend on Him and allow Him to flow like living water through us. Is it any wonder that it is called the *peace of God that passes all understanding which will keep our hearts and minds* in Philippians 4:7? Ultimately, the same peace that Christ had, the very peace of God, can keep us in any circumstance. We must recognize its availability to us through our vital union with Christ, yield ourselves to Him and His control and allow His peace to flow through us. It is the same with the other fruit of the

Spirit (each fruit being a character quality manifested in Jesus Christ). We don't "rejoice in ourselves" but we are to "rejoice in the Lord." It is not a matter of our joy but of His, so the joy of the Lord becomes our strength. The realization and experiencing of these truths is the essence of living the Christ-like life as we face our daily struggles.

Lord willing, I'll be in the pulpit the next Sunday, August 24th. Thanks for demonstrating the love of Christ to me in so many ways.

September 16th

This week has involved managing the usual effects of the chemo administered last week and the antibiotics given to clear the sinus infection. I am nearing the end of what I call the "down" cycle caused by the chemo. Usually by the end of the second week of the treatment cycle, the body begins what I like to think of as the "up" cycle during which you get stronger and feel better. When I think of this cycle of "downs" and "ups," I am reminded of what Solomon said in Ecclesiastes 7:14 that when we prosper, be joyful, when in adversity, consider, since God has appointed both. Here Solomon is observing that both prosperity and adversity are a part of every life. He also teaches what attitude each should produce in us: enjoyment and appreciation during the times of prosperity and discernment and learning in times of adversity (which might be distress, misery, injury or evil). In the good times, fully enjoy and make the most of them and in the bad times, realize and learn from them as from a teacher. Each has a part in our personal and spiritual growth and development. We can't and won't know until they unfold what we will experience and when. It is so easy to take the times of prosperity for granted, not really appreciating and completely enjoying them. But it is equally easy not to learn from times of adversity the important lessons of endurance, dependence, humility, obedience, correction, trust, sanctification, prayer, reliance on God's Word, discipline, direction and resting in the Lord - all of which are Scriptural purposes or benefits of our adversities. Also, in times of adversity, it is helpful to anticipate the times of prosperity as a generator of hope because the Word tells us, *Faith is the substance of things hoped for...* (Hebrews 11:1). Since a number of you have tried to convince me that I look younger, better, more handsome and more erudite (scholarly and learned) without my hair, I've been contemplating permanently keeping the skin-head look. Now if I can find a way to prevent all of the screaming from Barb whenever I mention it to her, I'll have it made!

I have now learned that a bald head is a happy head because we no longer have to face the hairy side of life and we are relieved of the following worries: turning gray, bald spots, root color, hair care products and preserving a lock of hair. So baldness is prosperity not adversity! I always heard that a bald head is like Heaven because it is a bright and shining place and there is no parting there.
I am eternally grateful for your prayers and support.

September 23rd

This has been a good week as I am gaining strength day by day following my most recent round of chemotherapy. I am scheduled for my next round of chemo beginning Monday morning. Lord willing I'll be in the pulpit tomorrow and I am eagerly anticipating bringing the message. I plan to preach the first of two sermons on the topic, "The Apostle Paul's Principal Mindset and the Apostle Paul's Mindset Principles." The idea for these messages came to me as I was meditating on some of the epistles written by the Apostle Paul and the frequently recurring themes which were Paul's constant mindset. His concentration on these themes enabled him to face difficulties, confront problems, strengthen himself through every experience and stay on course through the many ups and downs he faced. I went through all of the writings of Paul and made a list of his mindset issues, then when organizing them in a systematic way, I discovered they could be distilled down into six mindsets which are the subject of Sunday's message. The second message will deal with how Paul adjusted his focus, including both thinking and actions, to constantly establish and maintain these mindsets regardless of what he faced. By knowing and incorporating these same mindsets and using his methods, we should all be helped to have maximum effectiveness in becoming what Christ wants us to be and do regardless of the circumstances in our lives. A mindset is defined as a mental attitude or a fixed state of mind. It seems evident that our state of mind, as we go through the various experiences in life, makes a tremendous difference in shaping our responses and reactions as well as our attitudes, emotions and outlook.

So Lord willing, I'll see you all tomorrow in church and have the privilege of personally thanking you for your prayers and encouragement. You are the very best!
Love to all in Christ

September 30th

Yesterday I finished my fifth round of chemotherapy. I am always glad to complete the treatment week and the next week when the chemotherapy agents are attacking the cancer cells. They also attack good cells in the body resulting in a variety of unpleasant symptoms or possible complications. I am grateful for the medical advancements made during recent years which have provided better management of nausea, hiccups, cramping, fatigue, infection, discomfort, etc.

I concentrate on optimal thinking (knowing and facing the reality of any circumstance while factoring in God, faith, prayer, hope, Biblical solutions and practices, Biblically-focused attitudes and thinking) with focus on what is true, honest, just, pure, lovely, of good report with virtue and praise. We are told to continue to think on these things in Philippians 4:8. The control of our thoughts is so important because *As a man thinks in his heart so he is* (Prov. 23:7). Letting Christ live and flow in and through you is critical to this process, especially when the struggles or problems are the greatest or the circumstance the hardest. When our strength is ending, His is only beginning. Praise is always the ingredient for finding access to and experiencing God's presence. God promises that *He inhabits the praises of His people* (Psalm 22:3). The Hebrew word for *inhabits* in that verse has the idea of remaining, abiding, dwelling or staying put in a mindset of praise and gratitude. Focusing on the roses instead of concentrating on the prickly thorns helps lift the heart instead of further weighing it down.

Once when I was complaining to an insurance representative about escalating costs of the church's health care premiums, he mentioned that years ago when doctors performed a surgery, they would put a piece of rawhide in the patient's mouth, pour some whiskey on the wound and proceed to cut while the patient was fully awake. He suggested that if we returned to that state of practice, costs would decrease dramatically and become quite cheap. He then mentioned some of the advances made in recent years in modern medicine: diagnostics (CT, PET, SPECT scans, MRIs etc.), treatments (laparoscopic, micro and computer assisted surgeries, delicate and intricate arterial catheterization procedures, etc.), state-of-the-art hospital facilities and treatment centers, doctors trained in numerous specialties with ever-increasing knowledge and expertise, the proliferation of specialized drugs to control and cure diseases and infections as well as manage pain and ongoing research. All these offer hope for future successful treatments to improve both the quality and length of our lives. After saying that, he asked if I would like to go back to the rawhide or have the benefits of modern medicine and then added, "If so we will have to pay for it and all of these things are expensive." Believe me, I have thought about his words during my diagnosis and treatments and am glad we are where we are today. It makes it so much easier to look at some of the roses instead of the thorns and focus on an attitude of gratitude and praise. Recently, I have been reading the book of 2 Corinthians with great profit both as a source of encouragement and of understanding. Though I have studied it many times, God has provided fresh insights in the light of my current circumstances. God's word is like mining for gold. The more we dig, the greater the find of rich ore. The truths of God are like the multi-facets of a diamond with a reflection and application for every situation. How gracious God is to bring them into our lives at the times we need them most and to reveal them in such a meaningful way. Paul said to follow him as he followed Christ and added that the same comfort we find in the Lord enables us to pass it on to others. It includes being a human example, sharing our experience, and providing understanding, empathy, sympathy, guidance and strength as the ingredients of genuine comfort from God (1 Cor. 4:16; 2 Cor. 1:4).

Lord willing, I'll be preaching next week and have the privilege of delivering the second message on "Paul's Principal Mindset and Paul's Mindset Principles."

How about this, Barb mentioned that when I'm finished with my chemo, maybe I should keep my hair (or lack thereof) the way it is! See, God does work in mysterious ways.

October 7th

Good morning on this beautiful fall morning. Perhaps it would be better to wish you God morning instead of good morning because every morning is in reality a God morning. Regardless of the season or weather, it is one to be fully experienced and appreciated because of God's goodness. This has been a rough week. The numerous symptoms associated with the chemo's negative results on the body which I have previously mentioned have been strongly present this week. Although I used many remedies prescribed by my doctor, I had to weather the extreme fatigue and resulting discomfort. I was so weak and woozy one day this week I found myself toppling toward the floor. I managed to break the fall with my hands keeping my head from hitting the floor first. The cumulative effect of the chemo is taking its toll, making the symptoms more severe and harder to handle. Careful attention to my movement is a must. Some of the treatment cycles are easier to tolerate than others and I've found it impossible to predict which it will be. You can only be thankful for the easier ones and patiently endure the difficult ones. I found myself on numerous occasions during the week reading the blog which I posted last week to lift my spirits and focus my attention on the things I needed to be doing to help my attitude and channel my thinking in the right direction. It was a week that put those principles to the test in the crucible of life and drove me to practice what I preached. It is interesting how God so often has a way of doing that, isn't it? The good news is that the suggestions are good, but they must be worked into our lives as James suggests, *A doer of the word and not merely a hearer only, deceiving our own selves* (James 1:22). So last week's blog turned out to be prescient of what I would have to face during this second week of my fifth treatment cycle. As next week approaches, I eagerly look forward to my body's rebuilding process which means fewer symptoms and much more energy.

Thank you for your many prayers. I assure you they have sustained me throughout this past week, and I can't conceive what it would be like without them. Lord willing, I'll be preaching next Sunday. I'm really looking forward to seeing you all then.

The other day I came to a definite decision about my wardrobe while I remain hairless - I will never wear a turtleneck sweater because as the turtleneck collar extends to my bald head, it makes me look too much like a roll-on deodorant stick!

October 14th

After having a bad week last week, I started chilling and had a fever early this week. My doctor ran tests to determine if I had an infection and also checked my blood cell levels. He concluded that I was suffering from a viral infection but that my blood cell counts were good. So I have been fighting a cough and congestion most of this week. Monday the doctor will determine if I will have my sixth and final round of chemo. If I'm not completely over my viral infection, the week of chemo will have to be postponed. I had hoped to preach tomorrow but will not be able to do so. Please pray that I will recover quickly from this viral infection and that it will not develop into a secondary bacterial infection. The good news is that my white cell count revealed that my immune system should currently be strong enough to fight this off. I am getting ever so close to finishing all my rounds of chemotherapy, and I'm eagerly anticipating completing that final treatment cycle. All things work together for good to those who love the Lord and are the called according to His purpose (Romans 8:28). God doesn't promise in this verse that all things are good but that He will make all things *work together* for good. Somehow He will use this latest setback accordingly.

There is a silver lining in my recent loss of all my hair - I was able after so many years to throw away my Head and Shoulders shampoo. Folks have been asking what I'm using now - Mop and Glow! Thanks for your prayers. I hope to see you very soon.

October 21st

What a wonderful time of the year it is with all of the magnificent signs of fall in full evidence - the beautiful multicolored assortment of leaves on the trees, the freshly dropped leaves coloring the ground, the crisp cool autumnal weather with frosty mornings and the general feel of fall in the air. It is important to take the time to fully enjoy and appreciate each day given to us by God and make time to notice all the nuances of people, places and things in our lives.

Consider Psalm 118:24, *This is the day which the Lord has made, we will rejoice and be glad in it.* We are encouraged to **this** day rejoice in the Lord. To rejoice is to experience real joy because the Lord is with us and ultimately everything will turn out alright. This Psalm makes a good motto for each day. This day and every day find your joy in the Lord in spite of illness or unpleasant circumstances. It may seem difficult at first, but a joyful mindset will bring peace and calm. In John 15:11, Jesus tells us that the very words He spoke should bring joy. God's Word is that source of joy, strength and comfort. Meditate on it for a soothing balm for your soul. John 16:22 records Jesus words, *Your joy no man takes from you.* Allow nothing to rob you of that joy! Then verse 24 admonishes us to ask in order to receive that our joy may be full. Ask for what you need, for healing, for relief from pain, for comfort, for direction or for hope. Then rejoice as the answers come. Nehemiah 8:9-10 tells the people after a harrowing national crisis, *Neither be grieved, for the joy of the Lord is your strength.* Psalms 16:11 teaches He will show us the path of life and that *in His presence is fullness of joy.* What better place to dwell then in his presence! Philippians 4: 4 tells us that we are to *rejoice in the Lord always and again I say rejoice.* Joy comes only from the Lord. Lift your eyes above illness, pain, problems, disappointment and hopelessness and behold Him who alone can fill you with joy.

If these are not adequate reasons for which to rejoice and be glad, consider the Psalmist's emphasis on our personal choice in the matter. He said, ***We will*** *rejoice and be glad in it.* It is in our hands, we choose to rejoice and be glad or choose not to. We have only to put it into practice daily and see what a difference it will make.

Lord willing, I will be preaching tomorrow a.m. in both services. My viral infection is gradually improving with no further complications, I will begin my sixth and final round of chemo on Monday. Thanks for all of your prayers and please continue to pray that I will not have complications. By the way, my hair is beginning to grow back. I thought it might grow back thick, curly and black as it was in my youth, but alas, it is thin, gray and straight. Oh well, I will rejoice and be glad anyway and call myself "the silver eagle" instead of "the bald eagle."

October 28th

It is 4:00 a.m. Today's blog will be somewhat brief mainly because of the hour. I completed my sixth round of chemotherapy yesterday and was very glad that my viral infection had resolved and did not further delay my treatment schedule. The week of chemo went reasonably well and I am now getting ready for the remaining weeks of this treatment cycle, meaning the aftermath of the teardown and rebuilding going on which I have mentioned in previous blogs. One of the complications of the chemo is sleep disturbance. Normal sleep patterns are interrupted and you can be awake for long hours at night. I sometimes joke that I often get up at 4:00 a.m. because I'm wide awake. But having not slept wears one out. Such is the case today. I am getting ready to go to bed because I haven't been to sleep yet. Usually when that happens, I finally manage to get to sleep in the early morning. Looking on the bright side of the subject, you can get a lot done during those sleepless hours if you're feeling up to it. I often go in my office at home and work while Barb sleeps. From my reading in Romans and 1st and 2nd Corinthians, I have found much encouragement and support. God has been wonderfully ministering to my heart and I am eager to share with you what I've learned through the process. I am ever so grateful for your prayers and love.

November 4th

This has not been a good week. I began experiencing discomfort on the right side of my chest and back and soon had sores covering the right side of my chest extending under my arm and continuing across my upper back. Based upon my symptoms, I suspected it was shingles, which the doctor confirmed when I saw him early the next morning. I figured out why they call them shingles - because it feels like somebody took 16 penny nails used to hold shingles to a roof and pounded them into my body. They are quite unpleasant! I'm taking a variety of meds including pain killers to keep as comfortable as possible, and I'm grateful for every one and the relief it affords. Of course this hit when my immune system was at its lowest. I am extremely anxious for my immune system to improve so that I will be able to overcome this latest setback. Going through this ordeal has triggered flashbacks of having chickenpox as a child and I can't seem to remember much positive about that. I remember constantly asking my mother how much longer this was going to last and never being satisfied with her response. Please pray that my immune system will quickly strengthen, that I will have a quick and complete recovery and that the Great Physician will soon complete His healing work in me.

There are some positives to consider through this latest setback. I'm grateful it happened during the last chemo treatment instead of earlier on; I'm grateful for the meds available to provide palliative care for this condition; I'm grateful that the Great Physician promises to be with me through everything I must face and to be an ever present source of comfort and strength as my High Priest who can be touched with the feelings of my infirmities. I'm grateful for the faithful prayers on my behalf as *The effectual fervent prayer of a righteous man avails much* according to the Bible.

November 11ᵗʰ

Few people could complain about the weather we enjoyed earlier this week with temps in the mid-70s. For this second week of November, it was mighty nice for a change. The refreshing warmth and brightness of the sunshine is so uplifting after several days with overcast dreary skies. It is not a coincidence that the Son of God is called Sun of Righteousness as one of the many metaphors used in Scripture. In fact there are exactly 365 separate names and titles for our Lord given in the Bible, one for each day of the year. It is quite a devotional study to examine each of these names and titles and their applications as they relate to God's Son.

Although there are probably some twenty-five parallels between the sun and Son, consider this important teaching. The sun with its remarkable warmth, light and brightness is always there whether visible or not. During those days when the clouds block the sunshine from our view leaving us with darkened dreary cloud-filled skies, the sun is still very much present. You can board a plane on such a day, climb through the thick cloud cover and suddenly experience the burst of sunshine as you soar above those clouds. That is how it can be for a child of God. Circumstances can make life seem overcast and dreary. It is as if God's presence is far removed from us and we don't sense or feel His closeness. Many of the Psalms are reflective of this theme. Men of God experienced dark days or periods of defeat or sorrow. As they expressed their anguish and cried out to God to manifest His presence to them, they soon realized that He was always there. They just needed to look above the clouds and be reminded to experience the fullness of His presence. So when He seems far removed, pray until the sun breaks through. In Psalm 22, the Psalmist suggests praising the Lord as the way to roll back the clouds in your life to experience God's presence when he states, *God inhabits the praises of His people.*

Dealing with shingles has been a difficult experience. Facing the usual after-effects of the chemotherapy has been compounded by the pain and problems associated with the shingles. Some days have been cloud-filled and dreary, but thank God, I realize that He is ever-present and on those days I must be vigilant in rolling back the clouds through prayer, the Word and praise until the sun (Son) bursts through. The shingles are gradually improving and I am slowly feeling better. Please continue to pray for me. I hope to be back in the pulpit very soon. Meantime may the sunshine of His presence fill your life today.

November 18th

On this Saturday, my writing will be unusually brief. Although the shingles are improving daily, I still have lesions under my right arm which make it both difficult and uncomfortable for me to do much typing. I'm planning to be in the pulpit for both services tomorrow a.m., Lord willing, preaching a Thanksgiving sermon entitled "The Love Equation: Greater Forgiveness = Greater Gratitude." This is a message I'm particularly anxious to bring because of its timeliness and relevancy in our lives. Please continue to pray for me. I will be having some tests after Thanksgiving to assess the effectiveness of my chemo treatments. I'll look forward to seeing you all tomorrow. You may have trouble recognizing me because I now have so much hair.

November 25th

Happy Thanksgiving! I hope you had a wonderful holiday with lots of good food and fellowship. All of my children and grandchildren were home. It is always a special occasion when we can all get together and enjoy each other's company. My recent bout with shingles has been an unexpected setback which has been both long and difficult. Progress has been slow with my recovery taking longer than I would have liked. Last Sunday after preaching both services, I was extremely weak and tired and experienced severe fatigue much of the week. Clearly I underestimated my strength level at the time and have decided not to preach tomorrow. Lord willing, I'll have regained my strength and be back in the pulpit next Sunday, December 3rd.

People often ask "why" when disasters or even mild disappointments occur. There are no satisfying answers to that "why." Unexpected incidents in our lives may be unplanned by us but they are never unexpected by God. Virtually every Bible character's life was filled with unexpected incidents including Adam, Abraham, Isaac, Jacob, Joseph, Moses, etc. The list includes all except Christ. The best way of viewing these incidents is Romans 8:28, *And we know that all things work together for good, to them who love God, who are the called according to His purpose.* Joseph had the proper perspective of this verse regarding his circumstances when mistreated by his brothers which resulted in his difficult experiences in Egypt when he said, *You intended it for evil, but God intended it for good.* Remember every such incident may not in itself be good, but God's promise is to make it WORK TOGETH-ER for good. Now how can you beat a promise from God like that!

December 2nd

Good morning on this wintry white Saturday morning. This has been another difficult week. I suffered unrelent-ing pain from the shingles but my doctor prescribed new medications which have alleviated much of the discom-fort. Thursday night I spiked a temperature and went to the emergency room for tests and treatment. I did not have pneumonia but have a bronchial infection. The doctor pre-scribed antibiotics and a cough syrup and sent me home to rest, which I have had no trouble doing. Today the fever is gone and I am beginning to feel human again. So all in all, from a human perspective, it has been a less than stellar week. But whenever I go through rough times I think of the suffering of my Savior on the cross. Seeing some of the vets in the VA hospitals after being severely wounded in Iraq or Afghanistan makes me realize that my suffering or discomfort is minor in comparison.

I have been reading again in the book of 2 Corinthians where, in chapter one, Paul reminds us that in difficult times God comes alongside us. He often brings someone else alongside of us who is also going through hard times so we can be there for that person just as God was there for us. Therefore, no times of difficulty are ever wasted because His healing comfort is made available to us and then through us to others. In fact, Paul mentions that the willingness to endure hard times as well as enjoy the good times provides us assurance that we are going to make it. Later in the chapter, he mentions that God had rescued him and adds He will do it again for us. He will rescue us as many times as we need rescuing. His report was that he had come through with his conscience and faith in tact and could face the world and other believers with his head held high because God had remained faithful to him and without compromise kept His promise. God's promises are stamped with the *yes* of Jesus. He has promised, but we must answer with a *yes* of belief and acceptance that not one promise will fail. We know then that God's *yes* and our *yes* together are behind what we preach and pray. Finally, God affirms us with His spirit, stamping us with His eternal pledge that He will complete in our lives that which He has begun. Wow! What more could you ask for than these powerful assurances provided by God in 2 Corinthians chapter one? Please take the time to read and review this great chapter. I'm sure it will be as much of a blessing to you as it has been to me.

I covet your prayers that I might regain my strength quickly from these last couple of setbacks following my recent completion of my chemo treatments. Pray God will renew my strength like the eagle that I might be able to run and not be weary and walk and not faint (Isaiah 40:31).

In light of my circumstances this week, I will not be preaching tomorrow morning, but rather taking the opportunity for rest and recovery. I'll hope to be able to preach next Sunday. Again, thank you for your many prayers and loving support.

December 9th

I am continuing to recover from my double-barrel set-back of the respiratory infection and shingles from which, thank God, I am slowly improving. I am rejoicing that my post-treatment tests for cancer came back normal, indicating my chemotherapy was successful. Now I face the tasks of strengthening my resistance and regaining my stamina. Please continue to pray accordingly and be aware that I am so grateful for all of your prayers on my behalf throughout my entire treatment process. Truly prayer changes things. Lord willing I will be preaching in both services tomorrow a.m. I'll be looking forward to seeing you then.

December 16th

Good morning on this beautiful unseasonably warm Saturday. I am continuing to recover from my shingles and respiratory infection. Monday I am scheduled for another chest x-ray to ensure that the lungs are clear. I am slowly recovering my strength and the lesions on my chest, side and back are gradually improving.

My recent bout with shingles has reminded me of the importance of patience, especially the teaching of Romans 5:3-5, *And not only that, but we also glory in tribulations, knowing that tribulation produces perseverance; and perseverance, character; and character, hope. Now hope does not disappoint, because the love of God has been poured out in our hearts by the Holy Spirit who was given to us.* So patience is produced (worked out, render one fit for) by tribulation (affliction, suffering, difficulties). What is patience? In the New Testament it is the characteristic of a man who is not deterred from his deliberate purpose and loyalty to his faith and piety by trials. From such patience comes character (proof of character under trial) and hope (expectation of God producing good) because the love of God is poured out by the Holy Spirit in our hearts. Please take special note of the role of the Holy Spirit in the process. This confirms Galatians 5:22-23 where it includes patience as a fruit of the Spirit. It also correlates with Luke 8:15 listing patience as the product of a good heart and James 1:3 where it is associated with the testing of our faith. God knows how much most of us need patience (I certainly do.) and shows us the pathway to obtain it. Remember that Romans 2:6-7 promises God's reward for patience which is the incentive to let the process work God's purpose in our lives, not only for our good but for God's glory as well.

Tomorrow we have our Christmas musical drama and, Lord willing, I'll bring the closing comments to wrap it up. See you then.

December 23rd

Good morning on this Christmas weekend. I would like to wish each of my readers a wonderful Christmas filled with the presence and purpose of Jesus Christ. I so appreciate your prayers and expressions of love and concern during my chemotherapy. Yesterday I had a CT scan of my chest as a follow-up to the x-rays taken earlier. I do not yet have the results and will share them when I do. I'm looking forward to spending some time with my children and grandchildren during this holiday season and hope you will have a blessed celebration also. I hope to preach this weekend and to see you in the services. That will be a wonderful Christmas present for me.

December 30th

Good afternoon. It is Sunday afternoon and I'm posting a brief blog as a follow-up to last week's blog. The CT scan was fine, no pneumonia or other significant problems showed up in the chest. I'll see the doctor for a follow-up appointment later this week. Happy New Year to all.

January 6th

Good morning on this 6th day of the New Year. I'll begin with an update of my condition. I'm slowly regaining my strength from my recent respiratory infection, shingles and the chemotherapy treatments. My recovery is proceeding at a slower pace than I expected, but thank God there is improvement. I've had some swelling in my feet and my doctor is running tests to better evaluate the situation. I shared in my last blog that the respiratory infection has cleared up as shown in the CT scan. Please continue to pray for my continued progress in regaining my stamina, healing of the shingles, resolution of the swelling problem and, of course, that I will be cancer free. Thank you so very much for your concern and prayers which have been so vital in my treatment and recovery. It has been so good to be back regularly in the pulpit for the last month. Thank you for your faithfulness in supporting me.

January 13th

I continue to undergo tests to determine the cause of continuing symptoms. So far all of the tests have come back as normal. I had more tests yesterday and will consult an infectious disease specialist on Tuesday. Thank God I am beginning to feel a little better. It appears that I am suffering from a low- grade infectious process in my body. I'll let you know when all of the tests and consultations are finished and we have definite answers. I am planning, Lord willing, to speak in both a.m. services tomorrow morning and hope to see you there.

January 20th

I have continued to have a low-grade infection which has proved resistant to drug therapy. It especially affects my energy and stamina. Though I have improved, I am not yet well. Hopefully, my latest treatment will be successful. Please continue to pray with me about this need and, Lord willing, I'll be in the pulpit tomorrow a.m.

January 27th

I continue to struggle with the pain from the shingles which is decreasing ever so slowly following the conclusion of my chemo. My weak immune system and severe shingles have combined leading to a very slow recovery. All of my recent medical tests have come back negative and my low-grade infection has slowly improved. The infectious disease specialist did not think that it was caused by the organism that showed up in an earlier culture. The recent episode of blotches on my face has cleared up with steroid treatment this week. I continue to covet your prayers for renewed strength and resolution of complications.

Lord willing, I'll be preaching the third and final sermon in the series, "So Great Salvation," tomorrow a.m. I look forward to delivering that message and seeing you in the services. Thank you again for all of your faithful prayers.

February 3rd

Hello on this cold winter Saturday. I continue to slowly

recover and am gradually gaining strength. I'm hoping there will be no more setbacks of infections, relapses or complications. I am trying to limit encounters with people as there is much illness during this flu season. An intestinal illness affected our staff in the church office and various family members have suffered from respiratory ailments. Folks have been thoughtful to stay clear of me when they are sick and I am very appreciative. I am rigidly following my post-treatment diet and am beginning a light strengthening regimentation. The shingles continue to slowly improve but still make their presence known. I continue to find much encouragement from God's Word on a daily basis and am blessed by your continuing prayers and concern. Tomorrow's sermon is "Peter's Prescription for Getting Along with Others." I hope all of us will be able to make it, Lord willing.

February 10th

I continue to gradually improve in strength and stamina. Each week shows some improvement and my wife tells me that it shows in my preaching week by week. For this I am very grateful. I realize that these improvements take time and that realistic expectations and patience are necessary ingredients of my recovery. Scripture teaches that tribulation produces patience and hopefully I am gaining more by going through this process. Thank you for praying for my complete healing and restoration. Lord willing, tomorrow I will preach part two of the series, "Peter's Prescription for Getting Along with Others," which will focus on like-mindedness, compassion and tenderheartedness. I hope to see you then.

February 18th

It is Sunday afternoon and I am publishing my blog one day late. In spite of frequent attempts yesterday, I was unable to get through to my blog page until today. Ahh...technical difficulties, the byproduct of this wonderful computerized world we live in! I continue to make measured progress in my recovery every week. Although the progress is taking longer than I had expected, I've been told this is often the course it takes. It would be easy to look on the negative side of things, but that would be a mistake. I am grateful that I am neither going backwards nor standing still; slow progress is still progress and every week I show more strength and stamina. Thank the Lord for His provision and marvelous grace. My focus must stay upon how far I've come, not upon how far I have yet to go. God bless you for your concern and prayers. They are treasured blessings.

March 3rd

Blogger was changing over to a new format using Google and it refused to admit me until the changeover was complete. It seemed strange not to do the blog since I have now been doing it faithfully for many months. At last, all of the changes have been made and, hopefully, I'll have no further problems in posting my blogs.

Each week I continue to gain strength and am grateful for the progress. The severe case of shingles continues to slow-llllllly improve. No, the word slowly is not a typographical error but is a reflection of the speed of recovery. I am doing some exercise to increase my stamina and regain some much-needed aerobic strength after being inactive for so long. Again I find the key word is patience in this process. I have always had a tendency to do too much too soon, but now not rushing the process is all important to avoid setbacks. Thank you again for faithfully praying for me. Your prayers have been and continue to be so vital. James reminds us, *The effectual fervent prayer of a righteous man avails much.* Tomorrow, Lord willing, I'll preach the fourth message in the series on "Peter's Prescription for Getting Along with Others." I hope to see you then.

March 10th

I continue to gradually improve and find each week a little better than the week before. Planning activities, avoiding germs, strengthening exercises, controlling diet and limiting stress producers are all critical factors in my continuing recovery. Of course, the most important of all is the work of the Great Physician throughout the process. It is essential to begin each day by filling your mind with the encouragement and inspiration found by reading God's Word. It is God's voice speaking directly to our mind and heart each day. Then continuing God consciousness throughout the day brings the Lord into our thoughts, attitudes, motivations and actions. He provides the ultimate attitude adjustment by applying Scripture to our circumstances. God knows exactly what we need and will provide it if we allow Him to do it. His continuing strengthening and encouragement are available throughout the entire day regardless of what we face. He is our *ever-present help in time of trouble.* Prayer is our personal hotline to Heaven. Through it we can count and share our blessings with the Lord, present our needs, pour out our feelings and concerns, seek His presence and help as well as intercede for others and their needs. Counting and sharing our many blessings reframes our problems and praying for others helps us refocus away from those problems. What a powerful combination, God's Word allowing God to speak to us and prayer allowing us to speak to Him.

Please continue to pray for the following things: that I will be cancer free, that I will have no further complications, that my shingles will be completely healed and that I will regain my strength and stamina. Thank you for praying for me and my needs.

Tomorrow's Sermon is Part 5 of the series, "Peter's Prescription for Getting Along with Others." It will be a very practical presentation on not returning evil for evil. Lord willing, I'll see you then.

March 17th

I have continued my pattern of gradual improvement this week and feel a little stronger and mentally sharper. I continue to improve in both my strengthening and stamina-increasing exercises. Recently, I have been reading in the Gospel of John, and this morning I read chapter 11, the passage about the raising of Lazarus from the dead. Of special note was when Jesus said that Lazarus' sickness was for the glory of God and that their faith might be increased by giving them new reasons for their belief. I know that my experiences of the last months have influenced the faith of many others in addition to my own. Many of you have mentioned that these blogs have encouraged, taught and strengthened you and your faith. That is surely one way that this sickness has been to the glory of God. The glory of God is really the character of God and includes all that God is (omnipotent, omniscient, loving, unchanging, just, omnipresent, compassionate, etc.) and all that God is capable of doing. When those are in evidence, we can see the fingerprints of God. Many turned to Christ because of Lazarus and many believers had their faith "charged" and changed through his experience. It is often through the lives and experiences of others that our faith is influenced. Many of you have influenced my faith as I have seen the way you have faced life's trials. This is God's plan because our lives are the "Bible" that many will read.

As always, I thank you for remembering me in your prayers. Tomorrow, Lord willing, I'll be preaching another message in the series "Peter's Prescription for Getting Along with Others." I hope you'll be able to be there.

At this point in my recovery, I was able to stop using a stool for support as I preached and resumed my normal preaching routine. During Easter weekend I preached four times with no problems. In early May, I had an appointment with my oncologist for a six month checkup. All the lab work was normal and his physical exam revealed nothing remarkable. My strength continued to incrementally improve each month as did the shingles. I could raise my right arm to the level of my face and would describe the symptoms as more discomfort than pain. I continued on the path of progress and healing and was ever thankful for God's continuing work in my life.

I am happy to report that I continued to improve during the following months and now have yearly checkups. I have been in remission since October 2006.

If suffering does not have a purpose, it is random or meaningless. I have gathered Biblical principles about suffering which helped me to endure my cancer journey with the best perspective and attitude. I pray they will do the same for you.

Suffering increases awareness of the sustaining power and presence of God (Psalm 68:19).

Never underestimate the power of God's presence to see you through difficult circumstances. If you were alone without God being with you, imagine being in the lion's den with Daniel, in the fiery furnace with the three Hebrew children, a slave in Egypt with Joseph, in jail with Paul, on the battlefield with David, facing stoning with Stephen or in exile on Patmos with John. The Lord was with each one of these men in their individual circumstances. His presence provided protection, strength, comfort, help and hope to each of them. He will do the same for you.

Suffering refines, strengthens and perfects us (Hebrews 2:10).

The refining process separates the dross from the precious metal. Our trials of suffering help to remove the impurities from our life by developing our character, making us evaluate our priorities and showing us what should be most important to us. Our suffering can make us more sensitive servants of God. By having known pain, one can better understand and reach out to others.

Suffering prevents us from slipping or falling (Psalm 66:8-9).

Because suffering makes us weak, it forces us to be more vigilant and careful in our steps thus preventing a serious fall. Weakness makes us seek the Lord's strength when we falter in our hope and outlook.

Suffering allows the life of Christ to be manifested in us (2 Corinthians 4:7-11).

When Christ was on the cross, He didn't whine, rail or blame. If it is our desire to let people see God through us, it is His power in us that will accomplish our goal. Even under the intense pressure of suffering, He was filled with grace, mercy and compassion.

Suffering increases our dependence on God (2 Corinthians 12:9).

The Apostle Paul teaches that in our weakness, we can become strong. Weakness forces us to seek help from another. When we turn to Christ for that help, we learn to depend more fully upon Him for every moment, for every action and for every thought.

Suffering imparts the mind of Christ to us (Philippians 2:1-11).

In the book of Philippians, we are taught to have joy in spite of our circumstances, people, things or worry. This is accomplished by having the right attitudes of a single mind (doing God's will), a submissive mind (living for others), a sanctified mind (keeping the world and its things in perspective) and a secure mind (not allowing worry to overwhelm us). Philippians chapter 2 tells us that we are to *Let this mind be in you which was also in Christ Jesus*. Cultivating a single, submissive, sanctified and secure mind would be Christ-like thinking.

Suffering produces perseverance and hope (Romans 5:3-4).

As Christians we are told to sorrow not as others which have no hope (1 Thessalonians 4:13). Our faith should always be a source of strength in any situation because in Him we have faith, hope and love that never fade away. The ultimate outcome for any believer is victory. Whether we live or die, we are with Christ Jesus our Lord.

Suffering allows us to participate in the sufferings of Christ (1 Peter 4:14).

The word compassion comes from a root which means to "suffer with." The gospels mention that Jesus was filled with compassion, meaning He felt what others felt and suffered with them. When we suffer, we can better identify with, understand and appreciate Christ's suffering for us. (Philippians 2:5-8).

Suffering with faithfulness and endurance produces special rewards (2 Timothy 2:12).

Scripture says, *If we suffer with Him, we will reign with Him*. It also promises if we are an overcomer, we will sit with Christ in His throne. Now that is some promised reward!

Suffering produces the opportunity for others to demonstrate caring and generosity to us (Philippians 4:12-15).

Giving with generosity and possessing and showing mercy are two of the 19 major spiritual gifts listed in the New

Testament. Philippians 4 specifically identifies these two spiritual gifts as being associated with suffering. The merciful are blessed because they obtain mercy (Matthew 5:7). The flip side is that our suffering allows others to exercise the spiritual gifts of generosity and mercy toward us. Thank God for those who are there for us when we need them most.

Suffering produces discernment and teaches valuable lessons.

Teach me good judgment and knowledge: for I have believed your commandments. Before I was afflicted I went astray: but now I have kept your word. You are good, and do good; teach me your statutes. The proud have forged a lie against me: but I will keep your precepts with my whole heart. Their heart is as fat as grease; but I delight in your law. It is good for me that I have been afflicted; that I might learn your statutes (Psalm 119:66-71).

Here are specific things the Bible says suffering teaches us.

(1) Suffering teaches us humility and keeps us from pride (2 Corinthians 12:7).

(2) Suffering reminds us of life's brevity and death's inevitability (2 Corinthians 4:8-10).

(3) Suffering teaches us obedience and self-control (Hebrews 5:8).

(4) Suffering Helps us to put material things in perspective (Philippians 3:8).

(5) Suffering teaches us to be thankful and appreciative (1 Thessalonians 5:18).

(6) Suffering teaches us that life is not merely happi-
ness or personal fulfillment but can give honor and
glory to God and fulfill His purpose (John 9:1-3).

(7) Suffering teaches us patience (James 1:2-3).

(8) Suffering teaches awareness of others suffering in
the world (2 Corinthians 1:7).

(9) Suffering teaches us what is important in life (Job
21:7, 15).

Suffering and pain have a purpose.

Jesus experienced much pain and suffering even though
He was God in human flesh. Suffering and love are not
incompatible. The same pain that raises havoc in lives can
also be a gracious warning signal that something is wrong
and needs correcting; thus, pain may be good or bad depending on its extent, severity and duration. Many believe
that we would be better off were we to eliminate all pain.
Dr. Paul Brand wrote in The Gift of Pain: Thank God for
Pain, that he received a several-million-dollar grant to develop an artificial pain system in an attempt to assist sufferers of diseases such as leprosy and diabetes who were
in danger of losing fingers, toes and entire limbs because
of their faulty pain warning system. After many years of
work, repeated frustrations and millions of dollars spent,
Brand and his team abandoned their effort because a warning system for just the hand proved to be incredibly expensive, prone to frequent breakdowns and totally inadequate
to interpret the profuse sensations. He concluded what was
sometimes referred to as "God's great mistake" was actu-

ally a profound and complex warning system that the best in modern engineering and technology could not imitate.

Though pain is often quite unpleasant, it is that very quality that is so necessary to save us from destruction. His continuing work with lepers caused him to see pain as a divine gift to us to prevent a "painless hell." Lepers regularly were severely burned, wounded and even mutilated because of the absence of pain to warn them. It is that sensation of pain that warns us to remove our hand from a hot stove or withdraw our feet from broken glass. Without the warning system of pain, we would be unaware of the threat or process of injury or disease; yet the same pain that protects and helps us can be so devastating when we are ravaged by a serious disease process. Would we have been better off if our Creator had made us without a pain mechanism? Brand determined that without the overt unpleasantness involved in the pain process, the warning provided would be ignored or neglected. No wonder he co-wrote Fearfully and Wonderfully Made to express the profound amazement and wonder of the intricate workings of our bodies, including pain. How would we survive without it? It is like so many things possessing duality which can be tremendously beneficial or devastatingly destructive.

God promises to make all things work together for good to those who love Him and are called according to His purpose. How is that possible? How can God make bad things work together for good?

He promises that He will make all things work together **for good** to those who love God and are the called according to His purpose. How can God make all things work together for good? Note that he does not say all things in themselves are good, He only promises to make them work together for good. We observe many difficult and painful circumstances in our lives and wonder how God could possibly make these things work together for good. Recycling is a great example of this. When a tin can is discarded it begins to corrode, rust and becomes contaminated. It is scooped up and dumped into a truck to be taken to a recycling plant where it is melted down and recycled. Every original part of it is changed in the recycling process, and out comes a new can that is shiny, bright, clean and ready to be used. In much the same way, God takes the painful and difficult circumstances of our lives and transforms them through His recycling process. He fashions them after His purposes into a profitable, useful product (Romans 8:28). God has a way of bringing good things out of bad things. A thought to ponder: there could be no resurrection without the sufferings of Good Friday.

Based upon all of God's knowledge, He unfolds His eternal plan. Though the individual events are decided by the free choices of His creatures, God knows all possibilities and all possible outcomes. Based upon those choices, He then chooses the actualization of a specific plan based upon that knowledge. This concept is well illustrated in the life of Joseph. Although Joseph's brothers exercised their freedom of choice evident in their actions, God accomplished His purpose through their decisions. Many of those decisions were wrong and sinful, but God made them, though bad, to work together for good (Romans 8:28).

Consider the progression of events in Joseph's life: betrayed by his brothers and sold into slavery, falsely accused and imprisoned by Potiphar's wife, forgotten by his cellmate, elevated by Pharaoh, saved his family and nation –

all revealing God's providence through his ordeal.

Genesis records Joseph's instruction to his brothers regarding their decision: *Now therefore be not grieved, nor angry with yourselves, that ye sold me hither: for God did send me before you to preserve life. For these two years hath the famine been in the land: and yet there are five years, in the which there shall neither be earing nor harvest. And God sent me before you to preserve you a posterity in the earth, and to save your lives by a great deliverance. So now it was not you that sent me hither, but God: and he hath made me a father to Pharaoh, and lord of all his house, and a ruler throughout all the land of Egypt* (Genesis 45:5-8). *And Joseph said unto them, Fear not: for am I in the place of God? But as for you, ye thought evil against me; but God meant it unto good, to bring to pass, as it is this day, to save much people alive* (Genesis 50:19-20).

Suffering produces a broken and contrite spirit (Psalm 51:16-17).

Suffering shows us our vulnerability and helps us realize He is God and we are not. It humbles us so that we yield our will to His will and ways.

Suffering points us to the coming of Jesus Christ (1 Peter 1:13).

This verse says, *Wherefore gird up the loins of your mind, be sober, and hope to the end for the grace that is to be brought unto you at the revelation of Jesus Christ.* The revelation of Christ will be when He is revealed at His coming. Suffering makes us eager for Christ's coming to bring our deliverance.

Suffering is sometimes necessary to win the lost (2 Timothy 2:8-10).

I went to theological school with a couple who had a child born with serious medical problems. Although they were heartbroken about their baby's illness, they determined they would depend on the Lord to see them through. They made a conscious choice to live their lives in such a way through the crisis that they would be an inspiration and example of the love of Christ to those around them. One day their baby's specialist asked to speak privately with them. He noted that he had worked with them these many months and watched how they had handled their child's serious illness. He said, "You have been poised, thoughtful and filled with peace. How have you done it?" They welcomed his question and explained that they were Christians who trusted the Lord and believed He would see them through and make all things work together for good in their lives. After sharing their testimony, the doctor committed his life to Jesus Christ as he wanted to have in his life what they had. God used the sickness of their son to bring their doctor to a saving knowledge of the Savior.

Suffering allows us to comfort others who are struggling (2 Corinthians 1:3-11).

Perhaps no one can better understand and comfort another than one who has suffered through a similar difficult circumstance. I recall a fellow minister telling me of a member whose grief was severe. She had experienced great pain and suffering in the loss of her young child to a serious illness, but God saw her through and provided the comfort she needed. For the rest of her life, she sought out those who had lost a child. Parents reported no one helped them more or provided more comfort than this lady because she understood so well their pain.

Suffering draws us closer to Christ (Matthew 5:4).

Scripture says, "Blessed are they who mourn for they shall be comforted," in Matthew 5:12. The word comfort denotes that Jesus will reach out His loving arms and pull us close where we will be supported and comforted by Him. *Underneath are His everlasting arms* will become a personal reality to any who experience this blessing. Is it any wonder why those who experience His presence in this way are called blessed.

Suffering tests our spirituality, character and values by showing our reaction under pressure (Job 1:1-11).

Dr. James Stalker, expounding 1 Corinthians 4:1-5, shows that every person is in reality four people: (1) the person our acquaintances see, (2) the person our family and close friends know, (3) the person we see in the mirror and know ourselves to be (motives, true feelings) and (4) the person God sees and knows. The ideal is to have all four of these personages be the same with no hypocrisy. Suffering often precipitates the harmonization of the four by pressing us into the mold of the image of Christ by purging our character and clarifying our values.

Suffering brings more of the grace of God (2 Timothy 1:7-8).

God's grace is more than His unmerited favor. It is God's divine enablement that we become what He has chosen us to be and that we accomplish the works planned for us. That's why the Apostle Paul constantly opens his New Testament epistles to the churches with the words, *Grace and peace be unto you.* When he writes to individuals he writes, *Grace, mercy and peace be unto you.* He begins his letters with the prayer that God would give them grace. We need God's divine enablement to face the issues whatever they may be. Thank God for his unfailing grace.

Charles Haddon Spurgeon was caught in the middle of a terrible outbreak of the plague during his pastorate in England. He drove himself day and night ministering to the dying throughout the city. Exhausted, he collapsed into his chair in his office and told God he could not go on. As he sat at his desk, his eyes fell on the Scripture before him which read, *My grace is sufficient for you.* That Scripture reminded him that the power and presence of the Lord was within him and would rejuvenate his soul and body. He claimed that grace and went out into the streets and continued ministering until his job was done.

Suffering increases our faith (Jeremiah 29:11-13).

It increases our faith by driving us to the Word of God which is the source of that faith. It also increases our faith by showing us the reality of God's presence, power and promises. According to Job 3:11 suffering drives us back to the basics of our faith.

Suffering's tears will benefit all of Heaven (Psalm 56:8; Revelation 5:8).

God never wastes a tear of our suffering and sorrow. The Bible tells us God collects our prayers that will be poured out on God's altar and will provide a wonderful fragrance which will be aromatic for all of Heaven.

Suffering can produce an ultimate good, even bringing good out of evil (Romans 8:28).

Good and bad are relative terms. Our judgments about what is ultimately good or bad are often faulty. How do we know what is really good for us? Bad is, in reality, often good, or it leads to good, and vice versa. The following story is often told of an old man in a village. It illustrates the role our perceptions play in how we perceive events as good or bad.

Once there was an old man who lived in a tiny village. Although poor, he was envied by all, for he owned a beautiful white horse. Even the king coveted his treasure. A horse like this had never been seen before—such was its splendor, its majesty and its strength. People offered fabulous prices for the steed, but the old man always refused. "This horse is not a horse to me," he would tell them. "It is a person. How could you sell a person? He is a friend, not a possession. How could you sell a friend?" The man was poor and the temptation was great, but he never sold the horse. One morning he found that the horse was not in the stable. The entire village came to see him. "You old fool," they scoffed, "we told you that someone would steal your horse. We warned that you would be robbed. You are so poor. How could you ever hope to protect such a valuable animal? It would have been better to have sold him. You could have gotten whatever price you wanted. No amount would have been too high. Now the horse is gone, and you've been cursed with misfortune." The old man responded, "Don't speak too quickly. Say only that the horse is not in the stable. That is all we know; the rest is judgment. If I've been cursed or not, how can you know? How can you judge?" The people contested, "Don't make us out to be fools! We may not be philosophers, but great philosophy is not needed. The simple fact that your horse is gone is a curse." The old man spoke again. "All I know is that the stable is empty, and the horse is gone. The rest I don't know. Whether it is a curse or a blessing, I can't say. All we can see is a fragment. Who can say what will come next?" The people of the village laughed. They thought that the man was crazy. They had always thought he was a fool; if he wasn't, he would have sold the horse and lived off the money. Instead, he was a poor woodcutter, an old man still cutting firewood, dragging it out of the forest and selling it. He lived hand to mouth in the misery of poverty. Now he had proven that he was, indeed, a fool. After fifteen days, the horse returned. He hadn't been stolen; he had run away into the forest. Not only had he returned, he had brought a dozen wild horses with him. Once again the village people gathered around the woodcutter and spoke. "Old man, you were right and we were wrong. What we thought was a curse was a blessing. Please forgive us." The man responded, "Once again, you go too far. Say only that the horse is back. State only that a dozen horses returned with him, but don't judge. How do you know if this is a blessing or not? You see only a fragment. Unless you know the whole story, how can you judge? You read only one page of a book. Can you judge the whole book? You read only one word of a phrase. Can you understand the entire phrase? Life is so vast, yet you judge all of life with one page or one word. All you have is a fragment! Don't say that this is a blessing. No one knows. I am content with what I know. I am not perturbed by what I don't. Maybe the old man is right," they said to one another. So they said little. Down deep, they knew he was wrong. They knew it was a blessing. Twelve wild horses had returned with one horse. With a little bit of work, the animals could be broken, trained and sold for much money. The old man had a son, an only son. The young man began to break the wild horses. After a few days, he fell from one of the horses and broke both legs. Once again the villagers gathered around the old man and cast their judgments. "You were right," they said. "You proved you were right. The dozen horses were not a blessing. They were a curse. Your only son has broken his legs, and now in your old age you have no one to help you. Now you are poorer than ever." The old man spoke again. "You people are obsessed with judging. Don't go so far. Say only that my son broke his legs. Who knows if it is a blessing or a curse? No one knows. We only have a fragment. Life comes in fragments." It so happened that a few weeks later the country engaged in war against a neighboring country. All the young men of the village were required to join the army. Only the son of the old man was excluded due to his injury. Once again the people gathered around the old man, crying and screaming because their sons had been taken. There was little chance that they would return. The enemy was strong and the war would be a losing struggle. They would never see their sons again. "You were right, old man," they wept. "God knows you were right. This proves it. Your son's accident was a blessing. His legs may be broken, but at least he is with you. Our sons are gone forever." The old man spoke again. "It is always impossible to talk with you, you always draw conclusions. No one knows. Say only this: Your sons had to go to war and mine did not. No one knows if it is a blessing or a curse. No one is wise enough to know. Only God knows."

Many things in life can be used for good or bad. Cars can provide wonderful transportation or may be destructive in accidents causing dismemberment and death; should we remove all cars to eliminate all auto tragedies? Concrete provides convenient walkways and streets, yet people severely injure themselves on the hard surfaces; should we eliminate all concrete? Wood is useful in construction and as fuel but can also become a deadly club; should we eliminate all wood? Fire is good for warming, cooking, cleansing and lighting, yet it can rage in destructive fury; should we eliminate all fire? God has given us all of these things for our convenience and benefit; yet in the wrong hands or when used carelessly, there are painful consequences. If we want to derive the good from so many things, we must also tolerate the bad they can cause.

Suffering provides opportunity for God to demonstrate His power as evidenced in the raising of Lazarus (John 11:14-15).

According to James 5, *The effectual fervent prayer of a righteous man avails much*. God has four ways of answering our prayers for the sick.

(1) He sometimes miraculously heals.

(2) He heals using doctors, medicines and our own immune system.

(3) He gives us grace to live with the suffering and bear the infirmity (as he did the Apostle Paul with his thorn in the flesh).

(4) He performs ultimate healing by delivering us from our suffering and taking us to glory.

Suffering helps us experience the promises of God (Luke 21:36).

There are over 3000 promises in the Bible. Suffering believers often search out and claim these promises because of their circumstances and therefore experience the reality of their validity.

Suffering may prepare us for God's future purpose (Genesis 50:20).

Fanny Crosby wrote many wonderful Christian hymns. Tragically she lost sight in both of her eyes when, as a child, a solution was placed in her eyes through a terrible error which caused her blindness. She maintained a tremendous positive attitude in spite of the how that terrible occurrence impacted the rest of her life. She used her blindness to "see" what those who had normal vision did not see – the spiritual world. Her epitaph on her tombstone reads, "These Blind Eyes Now See."

Suffering results from many causes (1 Peter 2:21).

Human error, results of genetics and natural law, sin, environmental factors, evil actions by others, participation in the sufferings of Christ, chastisement, and according to the book of Job, the mystery of God and the universe are some of the reasons for suffering. Like Job we often don't know why particular suffering occurs.

Our suffering and pain may allow others to be blessed (Ephesians 3:13).

The Apostle John spent the late years of his life isolated on the Isle of Patmos. I'm sure his circumstances were far from his preferred final days, but while on that lonely isle he wrote the greatest prophetic book of the Bible, the book of Revelation which informs us of things to come. Imagine if that book had never been written.

Suffering prepares us to meet Christ (1 Peter 1:7).

Suffering people frequently have their ties to this world lessened causing them to yearn for something better when they will be free of disease and pain. When I have visited nursing homes through the years, folks would often ask me to pray that God would take them, telling me I'm ready and I want to go.

Suffering can turn you back to God (1 Samuel 5:6-7).

Many a sickness has opened people's eyes to the emptiness of their lifestyle and caused them to evaluate their lives in the light of eternity. Many of the testimonies I have heard were from people who experienced suffering that caused them to turn to God. Such was my own.

Suffering shapes us for special service to others (Genesis 45:5-8).

When Evangelist Bill Rice's daughter lost her hearing, he was devastated. But he searched for a way to turn that negative circumstance into a positive. He learned sign language so he could communicate with his little girl. Then he began teaching others sign language so that deaf people could be reached with the Gospel of Christ. Eventually, he opened the Bill Rice Ranch where thousands were trained in sign language, enabling them to begin ministries for the deaf in their churches. The ranch was opened each year so thousands of deaf people could "hear" the gospel. Bill Rice turned a tragedy into a triumph for Jesus Christ.

Suffering can be a source of honor for those who endure it (Philippians 1:29).

It can be a source of honor because it can:

(1) Demonstrate our loyalty to God (Proverbs 4:9-22).

(2) Manifest itself in better handling irritations while serving others (Mark 10:38-39).

(3) Build our character (Philippians 1:29-30).

(4) Become an example used to help others (2 Peter 2:21, 24).

(5) Help us to face reality because we know God is with us (Hebrews 5:7).

(6) Cause us to trust God for who He is, not what He does (Job 13:15).

(7) Prove our faithfulness and loyalty to God (Proverbs 4:9-22).

(8) Can bring glory to God (John 11:4).

Suffering helps the world to lose its attraction (1 Peter 4:1-2).

The army sergeant was barking out this order as he watched his squad setting up their tents, "Men don't drive those tent stakes too deep 'cause we're moving out in the morning." Because of suffering we are reminded that "This world is not my home, I'm just passing through. My treasures are laid up somewhere beyond the blue," as the song writer said.

Suffering enables us to empathize with the suffering on the cross (2 Corinthians 5:17).

Each Easter season in the Philippines, volunteers place themselves on a cross and imitate the crucifixion of Christ. It is a life changing experience because it enables them to identify with Christ's suffering on the cross. Empathy is the ability to feel another's pain and appreciate their suffering. The pain of Christ's cross was excruciating, a word from ex (out of or from) and crux (the cross). Experts tell us crucifixion is the most painful of torments, yet Christ endured it for you and me because of His love for us.

Suffering helps us to make reconciliation with others (Hebrews 5:8).

Katherine Marshall was the wife of Peter Marshall, who was then the chaplain of the United States Senate. She contracted tuberculosis and became bedridden for many months. During her long convalescence she was reminded of people she had wronged and struggled to make peace with each of them. She eventually got well but looked at her illness as a path to reconciliation with other she might have otherwise never contacted.

Suffering shows us where to find God through the fellowship of His suffering (Job 23:2- 5; Philippians 3:10).

The following incident reveals one man's close relationship to the Lord in his final days. A pastor received a call from a member of his church asking him to come to her home to visit her ailing father. When he arrived at her home, he was escorted into a bedroom and introduced to her father. After the daughter left the room, the pastor proceeded to sit down on a chair next to the head of the bed. Immediately the man said, "Please don't sit on that chair, sit over here instead," as he pointed to another chair in the room. He then explained that every day he spent time talking to the Lord in prayer. He added, "When I have a conversation with Jesus, I picture Him sitting in that chair next to me and pour out my heart to Him. That's why I asked you not to sit there." The pastor said he understood and when he finished reading a Scripture and praying with the man, he left the house. Several days later he received a call from the daughter telling him that her father had passed away and requesting that he perform his funeral. Later, when the pastor met with woman to make the funeral arrangements, she expressed surprise at how she had found her father. She said, "I had left him for a short time to go to the store and when I returned I went into the bedroom to check on him. I found he had died but his body was in the strangest position. He had pulled himself out of the bed and his head was resting on the chair next to the head of the bed. I wonder why he did that." The pastor explained what her father had told him during his earlier visit. He said that he was probably talking to Jesus when he died and he leaned out to put his head on Jesus' lap as he was being called home.

Stories of Inspiration

There are literally millions of stories about people who have survived cancer. Here are a few personal stories about those who have been close to me through my many years of ministry.

Marie's Story

Marie was being treated for colorectal cancer after a biopsy revealed she had a large malignant tumor. Her treatment consisted of both radiation and chemotherapy to shrink the tumor which was to be followed by surgery. Since the cancer had metastasized, her prognosis was guarded. During her chemotherapy she experienced nausea and weakness and constantly fought depression at the thought of having to wear a bag (colostomy) for the rest of her life. Her obsessive thinking about wearing the bag caused her to have so much despair she would withdraw into a world of silence during which she isolated herself from the rest of the family and brooded each day. Efforts by family members to cheer her up only made her more irritable and upset. But Marie experienced a positive transformation when a mutual friend arranged for her to meet a woman who had undergone the same treatment for the identical condition several years before. She was positive, strong and encouraging as she described how she had recovered from her cancer and adjusted to life with a colostomy bag. She talked about how grateful she was to be alive and cancer free and how much she enjoyed life every day. She talked about how the thought of what she would have to endure for the rest of her life initially tormented her until she decided that life with a colostomy bag was far better than leaving her husband and children behind and missing all the joys of watching her grandchildren grow up without her.

She mentioned that she would be glad to assist Marie in any way including helping her through her transition time after her surgery. Marie was so impressed by her new friend's attitude, she found her own attitude improving. she decided that she could choose to have an attitude of despair or choose to have an attitude of hope and acceptance. She decided that every day she would choose a positive series of thoughts rather than negative counterproductive ones and succeeded in doing so.

Today, Marie is cancer free and living a life filled with joy. She says every day is a gift and she is making the most of that gift. She adds that the colostomy bag is the price she pays to be alive and she works to accept it as a positive not a downer. She cherishes her time with family and friends and regularly serves with a cancer survivors group offering hope and inspiration to those needing it, especially those with colon cancer.

Helen's Story

Helen had a double radical mastectomy after mammography revealed a growth in each of her breasts and biopsies confirmed they were cancerous. The cancer was in an advanced stage having spread into her lymph glands. Although her surgeon said he felt confident that he had successfully removed all of the cancer, she worried that the doctor was wrong. After confiding in her doctor how concerned she was about having cancer still spreading undetected in her body, she accepted the recommendation that she see a counselor. She made an appointment with her pastor who related that he personally knew of twelve women in the congregation who had been treated for breast cancer and that all were doing well, some still cancer free more than forty years later. After hearing his recitation of several of their stories, she left his office with a peace and assurance. She determined she was going to practice the positive replacement principle of substituting positive thoughts about her recovery to supercede the negative ones. After learning that 85% of all the things we worry about never happen, she decided that she would not become a slave to worry now or in the future. She decided that she would not worry about a return of her cancer unless it did return – then and only then would she worry about it because then she would really have something to actually worry about. Today Helen is still cancer free seven years after her treatment. Whenever she is prone to worry, she reminds herself of her commitment to not waste her worry on a "what if" something happens scenario but substitutes a "wait until" it happens scenario instead. She has also learned to turn her worries into prayers and adds with a wry smile, "Why pray when I can worry?"

Bruce's Story

Bruce was in his early seventies when he experienced trouble urinating. He ignored his symptoms until he was unable to urinate at all. This crisis forced him to the emergency room in considerable pain. An urologist drained his bladder and later confirmed that he had prostate cancer. Having been incredibly strong and healthy all of his life, he was devastated upon learning he had advanced stage cancer. He chose what he thought was his best treatment option in consultation with his doctor. His recovery from his surgery was slow and difficult. When he returned home from the hospital, his family members took turns caring for him. Although his recovery was slow, he was able to return to his part-time job as a night watchman. A heavy smoker for

50 years, he decided that it was time to quit smoking after his doctor told him it would help his recovery. His long and difficult recovery made him concerned about his future. Although all of the cancer was not removed, he lived for many years with a decent quality of life. He enjoyed traveling, gardening and continuing his job. Many men fear incontinence after treatment but he did not experience further problems urinating. He was monitored on a regular basis after his treatment and enjoyed an active productive life. He lived into his early eighties and died following an emphysema episode, not from the cancer.

Jack's Story

Jack was experiencing a chronic cough which ultimately led him to his doctor's office for an examination. Tests confirmed a mass in the lung about the size of a small orange. He was scheduled for surgery to remove the growth. But the day of the surgery, Jack seemed to experience an amazing transformation. His pain was gone and he was feeling much better. He insisted that his doctor perform another test to confirm his need for surgery. The tests confirmed that the mass on his lung had shrunk from the size of an orange to the size of a pea. His doctor told him he had no plausible explanation for the change and the surgery was canceled. Eventually all traces of the abnormality on his lung were gone. Was it a mistake, a faulty test or a miracle? Who knows. Jack simply called it an answer to prayer.

There was a similar occurrence when I was a college student. One of the young ladies in our college class at church was diagnosed with a brain tumor. She too was planning to have surgery, and during the process her tumor disappeared. Those are the only two such cases I have known, and both certainly experienced amazing results. Perhaps someday we will have a better medical explanation for what happened, but in both cases, their doctors said they had no reliable explanation, and one simply called it a miracle. Sometimes there are amazing results, but these cases are very rare. Remember that God has several ways of answering our prayers for healing. He may miraculously heal as in Jack's case. Sometimes He heals through conventional methods - surgeries, medicines etc. He does not always heal, but gives us grace to live with and bear the infirmity. And sometimes He performs ultimate healing by taking us out of our pain and suffering by calling us home to Glory.

David's Story

David noticed a lump on his testicle. His doctor confirmed that the lump was caused by testicular cancer. Since Dave was in his 30s, he had convinced himself that he couldn't have cancer. But his doctor conclusively proved to him that his diagnosis was unmistakable. When he realized the fact of his condition, he cried. A personal friend, a doctor practicing in another state, comforted him by telling him that his chances of a full recovery were excellent if he submitted to treatment as soon as possible. After having an orchiectomy (removal of the testicle) David made a complete recovery. There was no recurrence after more than 20 years. Although he experienced a severe down time when he was initially diagnosed, he had a positive transformation of his attitude and outlook which continued during his treatment and recovery. David was thought by all who knew him well to be an infectious optimist, but the emotional swoon following his initial diagnosis was understandable because his diagnosis was so unexpected since he was young and healthy. He had a full recovery and remained optimistic about life.

Sarah's Story

Sarah was a young woman in her 30s when she developed symptoms which took her to her doctor's office for an examination. Her doctor told her that he needed to run a series of tests to rule out various serious conditions. After all the results were available, her doctor confirmed that she had advanced stage ovarian cancer. He explained that ovarian cancer tends to produce no early serious symptoms. As she began investigating details about ovarian cancer, she was alarmed at the treatment outcome statistics. She told her friends that she thought her cancer was a death sentence. Determined that she was going to fight her cancer with everything she could muster, she had surgery followed by chemotherapy. During her chemo treatments, she would watch as the chemicals flowed through the IV into her body and would picture the chemo drugs killing the cancer cells. She visualized the chemo acting like Pac Man gobbling up the cancer cells one-by-one until they were all gone. She took one day at a time during treatment and told herself that she could put up with anything for one day. When she was very sick, she had to shorten her time frame telling herself, "You can put up with this for one hour." This strategy saw her through her roughest days. She brought everything within her power to bear against her illness including sheer determination that she would live to see her children grow into adulthood. She demonstrated amazing resilience, desire and fortitude in attitude and action. Her determination was rewarded when she entered remission and remained so for the next

20 years. The attitude that she would be a survivor became a reality. She translated that attitude into both her outlook and her outcome. Against all odds she survived and became an inspiration to others including me.

Vernon's Story

One of my friends had a cancer battle story which has been a constant inspiration to me. His name is Vernon Brewer, the founder of the World Help organization which is dedicated to caring for those in desperate need around the world. Here is his story in his own words taken from one of his sermons.

They said, "We must operate immediately," and they sent me home to get my affairs in order. They said, "You probably won't survive this cancer," - it was very advanced. They removed a five-pound tumor off my heart and lungs. In that first surgery, they removed a portion of my left lung and my left diaphragm was paralyzed. It's still paralyzed to this day. They inadvertently severed the nerve to my vocal cords. For a year and a half I couldn't speak in an audible voice. They said, "If you survive, you'll never preach again."

Those were dark days: Eighteen surgeries and surgical procedures. A year and a half of chemotherapy ... in and out of the hospital for the better part of two years. At one point I had a catastrophe happen. The vein in my hand where I was receiving chemotherapy collapsed and they actually had to sew my hand to my side for a month - it was just one problem after another.

There is nothing joyful about cancer; it's a terrible disease. I remember when the doctor told me "You're going to have a year and a half of chemotherapy." My attitude was: 'Hey I can handle this, bring it on!'

You know it's going to be mind over matter, and the first time I received chemotherapy I said, "It's not all that bad. I think I can handle this." The next time I had received it, the disease had taken its toll and it was a little more difficult. The third time it was nearly impossible. The fourth time my wife and I walked up to the door of the doctor's office - I put my hand on the handle to walk in and I could not turn the handle. My wife said, "What's wrong," and I said, "I can't go in." She asked, "What do you mean?" I said, "I can't go in." My loving wife put her arm around me and prayed that God would give me grace to walk through the door. That was not joyful by any means.

I received a phone call from a pastor friend of mine while I was in the hospital. He asked, "What's God trying to teach you ... what sin is God trying to point out in your life?" That wasn't a good day for me and I was high on morphine, so I said, "Patience," and hung up the phone. I didn't want to hear that.

When I was going through chemotherapy, my neighborhood had a block party. We closed off the streets and everybody brought out their barbecue pits; everyone brought their own beer (it was bring your own bottle.) They were going to have a cookout and they invited us to come. My wife and I debated whether we should go, whether it would be a poor testimony to be where beer was being consumed, or what. I finally came to the realization that I didn't have any qualms about eating at a steakhouse where they were drinking beer, so why not have a steak in my front yard. Just because someone else is drinking beer shouldn't keep me from it. So I brought out my portable barbecue and brought out a big-ole 2-liter of orange crush so there would be no question about what I was drinking. And we went to the party.

My next-door neighbor was the superintendent of the county's public schools, and his wife, who was not a Christian, was undergoing eye surgery where she later lost sight in her eye. She said to me, "Vernon, how do you cope?" That's the question I was waiting for. I mean - she sent me a slow ball right down the middle. But no one was listening, so I pretended that the chemo had damaged my brain cells and said "What?" And she thought I couldn't hear well, so she yelled, "Vernon, how do you cope?"

Everybody at the party got real quiet ... it was like E.F. Hutton was speaking and they wanted to hear the answer to that question. Everyone was looking ... and I'm standing in front of my house, in front of my street, surrounded by 30 or 40 of my neighbors. I got to tell them what it's like to have Jesus Christ in your life and how you can face the trials of life with Jesus ... and that I couldn't imagine how anyone could face the problems of life without Jesus. Every one of my neighbors heard the Gospel that afternoon.

One day I wasn't doing real well ... I was losing the battle, so to speak, physically. The disease was taking over. I could tell I wasn't doing well because everyone whispered around me. You can just tell when you aren't doing well. I was depressed, and my wife said that we needed to get out of the house ... needed to go somewhere. She said there was a concert at the university tonight, and we needed to get tickets and go, and we did.

I was standing in front of the doors waiting for them to

open, and I found myself standing next to a friend of mine, Cal Thomas, a syndicated columnist for the Los Angeles Times ... perhaps you've seen him on Cable TV. What a voice crying out in the wilderness. He is a tall, lanky, dignified journalist. He turned to me and said, "Vernon be encouraged, I want you to know that I pray for you every day."

Now we throw those terms around a lot in Christian circles. But, he reached into his pocket and took out his Day Timer and flipped it to the back page where it said "Prayer requests." He showed me that my name was at the top of his prayer list. Now that ministered to me! He put his hand on my shoulder and said, "Now you be encouraged because God is going to heal you."

I walked in and sat down in the aisle seat and as the lights went dark, no one knew what I was feeling that night, but I was feeling like life was passing me by. I was having thoughts like - I'll never see my daughter's wedding ... there are so many experiences of life that I'm going to miss. Nobody understands the fear that I'm living with - nobody understands the uncertainty. I was feeling isolated, alone and scared.

Sandy Patty started singing, of all things, a song in Spanish, "Down the Via Delarosa walked my Savior" ... and a light came on. Wait a minute. There's someone who understands what I'm feeling. There's someone who understands what it feels to face death and isolation. There's someone who prayed, "Father, if it be possible let this cup pass from me, nevertheless, not my will but thy will be done."

I took great comfort in knowing that Jesus knew what I was going through, even if no one else did. And about that time something happened that I'll never forget. Sitting three or four rows in front of me was Cal Thomas. He got out of his seat, came back and sat down on the floor next to me and crossed his legs Indian style. He put one arm around me ... this dignified journalist in a business suit ... and held my hand. And I knew what had happened. I knew that God had tapped Cal on the shoulder and said, "Cal, my servant Vernon isn't doing too good. Would you go back there and put your arm around him and let him know I care." That was one of the most powerful moments of my life, to realize that Jesus cared.

Perseverance is not deliverance. We have a tendency to think that anytime a problem comes our way, all we have to do is pray and God will instantly deliver us from our problem. Don't get me wrong ... I believe in the power of prayer. I am here because God answers prayer. I will never forget November 25 when over 2000 Liberty University students prayed around the clock in the prayer chapel.

My dad called me on the phone one day and asked, "Son, how are you doing?" With my feeble whispery voice I answered, "Not so good Dad." He said, "I've got a verse for you; turn to it." He had me turn to the Old Testament to Isaiah 40:31, and he stated quoting it. "They that wait upon the Lord shall renew their strength; they shall mount up on wings as eagles, they shall run and not grow weary, they shall walk and not grow faint." I said, "Dad, I know that verse, you've heard me preach on that verse." *He replied, "Son, wait a minute - what do you need right now more then anything?" I said, "Strength." He answered, "Where do you get strength? Waiting on God. What does God have you doing right now? Waiting."*

(Following is a letter my dad wrote.)

Dear Son,

These past two weeks - there have been much searching and struggle for me. My heart is broken because of your pain and affliction. Even now while I am writing, I cannot hold back the tears. I've cried enough tears for the both of us, walking the floor and weeping through the night.

It has not been as difficult for us to accept the fact you have cancer, but I am having a hard time accepting the injury to your voice and vocal cords. Yet, I know that God doesn't make any mistakes and He is still in control and that Romans 8:28 is still true. However, I know what it means to think thoughts and to feel feelings and not be able to express them, and it hurts me deeply to think this could happen to you.

Would to God that I could bear this pain and affliction for you. It would be much easier for me to do. But, that would rob you of God's blessed purpose for you and the blessings He's going to build in you and the way He's going to use you with whatever voice He gives you.

In your personal odyssey of catastrophe I pray there would be this absorbing thought - God knows and feels your pain just as He did at the grave of Lazarus, and He weeps for you. Please take comfort knowing that His comfort is not insulation from the difficulty, but rather it is the spiritual fortification sufficient to enable you to stand firm, undefeated in this fiery trial that God is permitting you to bear. I just want you to know that I am bearing this with you and I've never loved you more.

Dad

Comfort for Terminal Patients

In spite of the best treatments, you may hear your doctor say, "There is nothing more we can do, you are going to die." It may or may not come as a shock, depending upon your awareness of your critical condition. Doctor Elizabeth Kubler-Ross worked extensively with terminal patients and observed that when they learned they were going to die, they usually went through several stages of grieving. The first stage is denial, "This can't be happening to me." Denial gives way to anger, which may be bottled up or expressed, "I'm angry this is happening to me. I don't want to die." Next comes bargaining, "God, if you let me live I'll do this and this and this. I'm going to find a way out." When the bargaining with God doesn't work, depression can set in, "I'm feeling hopeless, lost, devastated, sad and blue." For many, depression eventually leads to acceptance of the inevitable. The stages are not always in this exact order, may vary in duration and can be repeated. The physical process of dying may vary from person to person, but hospice and home care can provide direction, help and coping assistance. Jesus promises to be with us through it all to provide comfort and strength.

For the believer in Jesus Christ, there is unimaginable hope in the teaching of Scripture regarding the dying process and the life that awaits the Christian in Heaven. Jesus said, *I am the resurrection and the life; he who believes in me, though he be dead, yet shall he live* (John 11:25). Though our body may die, we will live on. Our body is like the house we live in. When we change residences, we leave one house and move into another. Although our address changes, we continue to live in our new location. So it is when we die, we move from our home on earth to our new home in Heaven. Jesus said, *In my Father's house are many mansions (residences); if it were not so, I would have told you. I go to prepare a place for you, that where I am, there you may be also* (John 14:1-2). The Bible not only compares dying with leaving one residence for another, but illustrates the process as slipping out of an old garment and slipping into a new better one. Our earthly body is subject to deterioration, disease and dying, but our heavenly body will be without any of those characteristics. Death comes as a release from suffering, pain and weakness. A cocoon is the first home of a beautiful butterfly, but it is left behind when the butterfly flies away. When we die, we go immediately to be with God. In 2 Corinthians 5:8 we read, *To be absent from the body is to be present with the Lord.* The Apostle Paul adds in Philippians 1:23, *Having a desire to depart, and be with Christ; which is **far better**.* These promises about eternal life are a reality because of what Christ did for us. His death, burial and resurrection and our trusting faith in Him provide the winning combination of deliverance and assurance.

The Psalmist beautifully illustrates the impact of the gospel on our life and walk now and forever when he wrote, *Even though I walk through the valley of the shadow of death, I will fear no evil for you are with me (Psalm 23:4).* Why does he say the *valley of the shadow of death* instead of just "valley of death?" Dr. Donald Grey Barnhouse, whose wife had just died, was driving to the funeral service with his children. He thought about how he could comfort his children in the loss of their mother. Suddenly a thought crossed his mind and he said, "Kids would you rather be struck by this truck sitting beside us or would you rather be run over by its shadow?" The children responded by saying, "That's easy Daddy, we'd much rather be run over by the shadow because shadows can't hurt us." He told them that because Jesus Christ took our sins upon Himself, died in our place on the cross and rose from the dead, He took our penalty and punishment as our divine substitute. So instead of being struck by the truck, we only experience the shadow. Indeed because Christ became sin for us who knew no sin, death has forever lost its sting and has no final power over us.

How Christ delivers us from the fear of death is further illustrated by M. R. DeHaan who used to raise bees. One day a bee escaped, swooped down and stung one of his boys. When one brother saw that the other had been stung, he jumped up and started running as fast as he could with Dr. DeHaan in pursuit. When he finally overtook his son, he asked why he was running. The boy replied, "Because I don't want that bee that just stung my brother to sting me." Dr. DeHaan then carefully explained that could not happen because the bee had only one stinger, and since the bee stung his brother, it had no stinger left and was powerless to sting him. What a wonderful illustration about what Jesus Christ did when He took the sting of death and removed it so that when we face death, the sting would be forever gone.

I have often heard people say, "I don't fear death, it is dying I fear." Note that in the twenty-third Psalm, the writer says that when he is going through the valley of the shadow of death, he will fear no evil because the Lord will be with him through the whole experience.

Peter Marshall, the former Chaplin of the U.S. Senate, illustrated what it was like to die in one of his messages. Here is an excerpt.

Sometimes people wonder what it's like to die. A little boy was dying. His mother and father had not told him that he had a terminal illness that would take his life, but the little fellow figured it out and finally asked his mother if he was dying. The mom knew that she could not conceal the truth any longer, so she turned away from him and whispered a prayer, saying, "Dear Lord, you know that my son needs an answer, please give me the wisdom to know exactly what to say." The little boy looked at his mother and said, "Mama, I'm afraid to die because I've never died before. What is it like to die?" Suddenly God gave her a wonderful thought. She said, "Kenneth, you don't have to be afraid to die. Do you remember a few years ago when you were younger and you would fall asleep on the couch watching television with Mom and Dad in the living room?" He said, "Yes Mama." She said, "When you fell asleep, you'd wake up in the morning in your own room and in your own bed safe and secure. When you fell asleep, your Daddy, with his strong arms, would pick you up and carry you into your room, put you in your own bed and tuck you in. That's what it's like to die, your body will simply go to sleep and the angels will come and carry you into the arms of the Lord Jesus Christ. So you don't have to be afraid, every-thing will be just fine. Son, that's what it's like to die." That satisfied the little fellow. He never raised the issue or asked about it again until God called him home. His mother's explanation had removed his fear and had given him great confidence that all would be well because it was under the control of the Lord Jesus Christ.

Sometimes we look at death as if it's a terribly negative thing, but the Bible clearly teaches that is not true. The Apostle Paul said that he had the privilege of seeing Heaven, and that it was so wonderful, he couldn't talk about it for 14 years. Now that he's mentioning it, he said that he was torn between two desires. On the one hand, knowing what waited for him in Heaven, he couldn't wait to get there; but on the other hand, because of the ministry and the desire to serve the Lord here, he needed to stay here and wait. Clearly he was torn between the two.

When a baby is inside the mother's womb getting ready to be born, imagine if that baby could talk. Maybe it would say something like this, "But I don't want to be born; I'm happy here; I've got everything I need right here in my mother's tummy. I have warmth, security, food and comfort. I want to stay here." And we might say to that baby, "But there's a whole new wonderful world waiting for you, and when you're born into it, you'll see what I mean." That's a good illustration of death and Heaven. We think that we don't want to leave this world because we're happy here, but God would say to us that there's a whole new wonderful heavenly world waiting for us when we are born into it through death. It's a place where there's no sin, no sorrow, no suffering, no heartache, no disease and no death - a place that He has prepared for us.

Finally, the Bible says that if we don't have the hope of life after death, then we are of all men most miserable. I couldn't give comfort to families or officiate at funerals if I did not believe these truths and was not able to offer the dying and their loved ones this hope.

When Rev. John Todd was a boy, he lost both of his parents and went to live with his aunt. He was so disappointed when his aunt did not come for him and take him to her home. Instead she sent her servant, a man whose name was Caesar. The two of them, together on Caesar's horse, rode the long distance to his new home. They rode through the darkness and coming out of the woods, they saw the house in the distance. A fearful John asked Caesar if he thought his aunt would be waiting for him. Caesar assured him that she was watching and was at that moment standing with a candle at the window eagerly waiting for him. When they arrived at the house, his aunt warmly welcomed him. She served him something to eat, tucked him into bed and sat by his side until he fell asleep. Now many years had passed, she was an elderly woman and he was a minister. She wrote him a letter expressing her fear of dying and asked him for advice. He wrote to her reminding her of that day so long ago when Caesar brought him to live at her home. He mentioned the fears and doubts he had and shared that seeing her standing in front of the window waiting and watching for him was such a comforting sight. He related how she so warmly welcomed him to his new home. He wrote that she had no reason to fear dying because, just as she waited to receive him home and gave him such a loving welcome, the Lord Jesus would be waiting and watching to give her the warmest of welcomes to her new home, Heaven. His letter allayed her fears and gave her great comfort and hope.

What a moment it will be when we meet Jesus face to face and reunite with loved ones who are waiting for us there. That will be...Heavenly.

I cannot close this chapter without sharing how you can have the assurance you need to be ready to meet the Lord. Billy Graham told the following story from the life of Albert Einstein. *The great physicist was said to be traveling by train when the conductor asked to see his ticket. After searching through his pocket, Einstein told him he had misplaced the ticket and didn't know where it was. The conductor assured him that it was alright since he knew him and accepted his word about having purchased one. As the conductor continued to pass through the car, he looked back and saw Einstein searching under his seat still trying to find his ticket. He went back and said, "Mr. Einstein, it is alright, I know who you are." To which Einstein replied, "Young man, I know who I am, but I must find the ticket because I don't know where I'm going."*

Many people don't know where they are going when they are facing death. Regardless of what we have done, God offers forgiveness for any and all of our misdeeds if we acknowledge our sins and ask His forgiveness. Scripture says, *If we confess our sins, He is faithful and just to forgive us our sins and cleanse us from all unrighteousness* (John 1:9). Believing in Christ is putting all of our personal trust in Him based upon what He did for us on the cross. It is wonderful to know who we are in Christ and where we are going because of Him. Thank God for the promise in Romans 10:13, *Whosoever shall call upon the name of the Lord, shall be saved.*

Conclusion

It is my fervent hope that this book has been a source of inspiration and encouragement to you. As I write these final words, I am saying a prayer for all of you who will read these pages. It is "May you experience the healing touch of the Master's hand. And may the Great Physician, our Lord Jesus Christ, give you grace, mercy and peace." Someone once said, "Do not be afraid of tomorrow; for God is already there." The song writer said it well when he wrote in the hymn, *I Know Who Holds Tomorrow:*

I don't know about tomorrow;
I just live from day to day.
I don't borrow from its sunshine
For its skies may turn to grey.
I don't worry o'er the future,
For I know what Jesus said.
And today I'll walk beside Him,
For He knows what is ahead.

Many things about tomorrow
I don't seem to understand
But I know who holds tomorrow
And I know who holds my hand.

Every step is getting brighter
As the golden stairs I climb;
Every burden's getting lighter,
Every cloud is silver-lined.
There the sun is always shining,
There no tear will dim the eye;
At the ending of the rainbow
Where the mountains touch the sky.

I don't know about tomorrow
It may bring me poverty
But the one who feeds the sparrow,
Is the one who stands by me.
And the path that is my portion
May be through the flame or flood;
But His presence goes before me
And I'm covered with his blood.

Many things about tomorrow
I don't seem to understand
But I know who holds tomorrow
And I know who holds my hand.

Comforting Scriptures

John 14:27 *Peace I leave with you; My peace I give unto you; not as the world gives, do I give to you. Let not your heart be troubled, nor let it be fearful.*

Psalm 56:3 *When I am afraid, I will put my trust in Him.*

Psalm 118:6 *The Lord is for me; I will not fear. What can man do to me?*

Luke 12:6-7 *Are not five sparrows sold for two cents? And yet not one of them is forgotten before God. Indeed, the very hairs of your head are all numbered. Do not fear; you are of more value than many sparrows.*

Psalm 46:1-2 *God is our refuge and strength, a very present help in trouble. Therefore we will not fear, though the earth should change, and though the mountains slip into the heart of the sea.*

Psalm 27:14 *Wait for the Lord; be strong, and let your heart take courage; Yes, wait for the Lord.*

Psalm 31:24 *Be strong, and let your heart take courage, all you who hope in the Lord.*

John 16:33 *...These things have I spoken to you, that in Me you may have peace. In the world you have tribulation, but take courage; I have overcome the world."*

Joshua 1:9 *Have I not commanded you? Be strong and courageous! Do not tremble or be dismayed, for the Lord your God is with you wherever you go.*

James 5:14-15 *Is any sick among you? Let him call for the elders of the church; and let them pray over him, anoint-*

ing him with oil in the name of the Lord. And the prayer of faith shall save the sick, and the Lord will raise him up; and if he has committed sins they shall be forgiven him, and the Lord will raise him up.

2 Timothy 1:7 *For God has not given us the spirit of fear: but of power, and of love, and of a sound mind.*

2 Corinthians 4:15-18 *For all things are for your sakes, that grace, which is spreading to more and more people may cause the giving of thanks to abound to the glory of God. Therefore we do not lose heart, but though our outer man is decaying, yet our inner man is being renewed day by day. For our light affliction, which is but for a moment, is producing for us an eternal weight of glory far beyond all comparison, while we look not at the things which are seen, but at the things which are not seen; for the things which are seen are temporal, but the things which are not seen are eternal.*

Psalm 25:16-18, 20 *Turn to me and be gracious to me, for I am lonely and afflicted. The troubles of my heart are enlarged; bring me out of my distresses. Look upon my affliction and my trouble, and forgive all my sins. Guard my soul and deliver me; Do not let me be ashamed, for I take refuge in You.*

Psalm 34:4, 6-7, 15, 17-19, 22 *I sought the Lord and He answered me, and delivered me from all my fears. This poor man cried and the Lord heard him, and saved him out of all his troubles. The angel of the Lord encamps around those who fear Him, and rescues them. The eyes of the Lord are toward the righteous, and His ears are open to their cry. The righteous cry and the Lord hears, and delivers them out of all their troubles. The Lord is near to the brokenhearted, and saves such as are of contrite spirit. Many are the afflictions of the righteous: but the Lord delivers him out of them all. The Lord redeems the soul of His servants; and none of those who take refuge in Him will be condemned.*

Psalm 147:3 *He heals the brokenhearted, and binds up their wounds.*

John 14:1-3 *Let not your heart be troubled; you believe in God, believe also in Me. In My Father's house are many dwelling places; if it were not so, I would have told you; for I go to prepare a place for you. And if I go to prepare a place for you, I will come again, and receive you to Myself; that where I am, there you may be also.*

Revelation 21:3-5 *And I heard a loud voice from the throne, saying "Behold, the tabernacle of God is among men, and He shall dwell among them, and they shall be His people, and God Himself shall be among them, and He shall wipe every tear from their eyes; and there shall no longer be any death; there shall no longer be any mourning, or crying, or pain; the former things have passed away." And He who sits on the throne said, "Behold, I am making all things new." And He said, "Write, for these words are faithful and true."*

1 John 5:14-15 *And this is the confidence that we have in him, that if we ask anything according to his will, he hears us: and if we know that he hears us, whatsoever we ask, we know that we have the petitions we desired of him.*

WHEN WEARY
Deuteronomy 33:7; Psalm 55:22
Psalm 73:26; Isaiah 40:31; Jonah 2:7; Matthew 11:28;
2 Corinthians 4:16

WHEN IN TEMPTATION
Psalm 1:1-6; Matthew 6:24; Luke 21:33-36;
Mark 13:33-37; Romans 13:13-14; 1 Corinthians 10:13;
James 1:12-25; Philippians 4:8

WHEN IN TROUBLE
Psalms 16, 31, 38, 40; 2 Peter 2:9

WHEN AFRAID
Psalm 27; Matthew 6:25-34; Matthew 11:28-30;
John 11, 17, 20; Romans 8; 2 Corinthians 4, 5;
2 Corinthians 12:9

WHEN DISASTER THREATENS
Psalm 20:6-9, 34; Psalms 118:5-9, 121, 126

WHEN BEREAVED
Luke 6:21; 1 Corinthians 15; 1 Thessalonians 4:13-18

WHEN DOWN
Psalm 91; Matthew 5, 4, 10-12; John 14:1, 16, 18, 27;
Romans 8, 28, 35-39

WHEN IN NEED OF COMFORT
Job 5:19; Job 11:16; Psalm 25:5; Psalm 30:5; Psalm
42:5; Psalm 103:13

WHEN DISCOURAGED
Psalm 23; 37:1-17; Psalm 55:22; Psalm 90:12-17;
Philippians: 4:4-7; 1 John 3:1-3

WHEN FAILED BY FRIENDS

Psalm 35; 41:9-13; Psalm 55:12-23; Luke 17:3, 4;
Romans 12:14, 17, 19

WHEN SICK OR IN PAIN

Matthew 26:39; 2 Timothy 2:3; Hebrew 12:1-11; James
5:11-15; 1 Peter 4:12, 13, 19

WHEN IN CRISIS

2 Timothy 1:7; Hebrews 4:16

WHEN ANXIOUS AND IN NEED OF PEACE

Psalm 1:1,2; Psalm 4:8; Psalm 85:8, 46, 107; Romans
5:15; Colossians 3:15; Psalm 107; Philippians 4:6;
1 Peter 5:6; Hebrews 13:5

WHEN IN NEED OF PRAYER

2 Corinthians 4:8-10, 16, 17;
Psalm 4, 6, 25, 42, 51; Matthew 6:5-15; Luke 18:1-14
John 17; 1 John 5:14, 15

Cancer Resource's Web Sites

American Cancer Society: http://www.cancer.org/index

National Cancer Institute: http://www.cancer.gov

National Cancer Institute Local Community: http:// www.cancer.gov/cancertopics/factsheet/Support/resources

American Medical Society: http://www.ama-assn.org/ ama

American Institute for Cancer Research: http://www. aicr.org

Cancer Supportive Care – Education and Information Resources: http://www.cancersupportivecare.com/education.html

Mayo Clinic Cancer Resources: http://www.mayoclinic. com/health/cancer-resources/MY01733

The Breast Cancer Research Foundation: http://www. bcrfcure.org/res.html

American Society of Clinical Oncology (ASCO): http:// www.cancer.net

American Lung Association: http://www.lung.org

American Pain Foundation: http://www.painfoundation. org

Association of Cancer Online Resources: http://www. acor.org

Susan G. Komen Breast Cancer Foundation: http://ww5. komen.org

Cancer Care: http://www.cancercare.org

Nexcura (Cancer Facts): http://www.usoncology.com/ hosting/nexcura/maintenance

Cancer Iowa (Iowa Cancer Consortium): http://www. canceriowa.org

Cancer and Leukemia Group (B): https://www.calgb.org

Care Pages: https://www.carepages.com

Children's Oncology Group: http://www.childrensoncol-ogygroup.org

Radiological Society of North America: http://www. rsna.org

Radiation Therapy Oncology Group: http://www.rtog. org

Oncology Nursing Society: http://www.ons.org

Be The Match (Bone Morrow Transplant Fascinators): http://bethematch.org

National Comprehensive Cancer Network: http://www. nccn.org/index.asp

National Coalition for Cancer Survivors: http://www. canceradvocacy.org

National Children's Cancer Society: http://www.chil-dren-cancer.com/Page.aspx

Healthfinder: http://www.healthfinder.gov

International Myeloma Foundation: http://myeloma.org/ Main.action

Leukemia and Lymphoma Society: http://www.lls.org

Locks of Love (Hair for Children): http://www.lockso-flove.org

MAMM (Women's Breast and Reproductive Cancer Resource): http://www.mamm.com/start.php

LiveStrong Foundation (Survivor Care):

National Children's Cancer Society: http://www.children-cancer.com/Page.aspx

National Coalition for Cancer Survivorship: http://www.canceradvocacy.org

National Comprehensive Cancer Network: http://www.nccn.org/index.asp

Gilda's Club: http://www.gildasclub.com/Default.aspx

Caring Bridge: http://www.caringbridge.org

Southwest Oncology Group (Designs and Conducts Clinical Trials): http://swog.org

North Central Cancer Treatment Group: http://ncctg.mayo.edu

Cancer Support Community: http://www.cancersupportcommunity.org/Default.aspx

Southwest Oncology Group (Designs and Conducts Clinical Trials): http://swog.org

North Central Cancer Treatment Group: http://ncctg.mayo.edu

About the Author

Dr. Mel Brown earned his doctorate in counseling from Northern Illinois University with special emphasis in Clinical Psychology and Marriage and Family Therapy. He holds degrees in Communications, Theology and Counseling and has supervised counselors at every level of experience.

He has pastored three churches and been in the ministry for over 50 years. During his ministry, he has delivered 15,000 sermons and authored 2,500 articles. He has received 20 academic and professional awards.

Dr. Brown is the author of The Minister's Instruction Manual and How to Choose the Right Mate, A Guide for Choosing Wisely.

He has been married to his wife Barbara for nearly 50 years and is the father of three, and grandfather of eight.

www.ingramcontent.com/pod-product-compliance
Lightning Source LLC
Chambersburg PA
CBHW071007040426
42443CB00007B/700